To my parents, for their unwavering support

Multivariable Analysis

Why do you need this book?

Multivariable analysis is confusing! Whether you are performing your first research project or attempting to interpret the output from a multivariable model, you have undoubtedly found this to be true. Basic biostatistics books are of little to no help to you, since their coverage often stops short of multivariable analysis. However, existing multivariable analysis books are too dense with mathematical formulas and derivations and are not designed to answer your most basic questions. Is there a book that steps aside from the math and simply explains how to understand, perform, and interpret multivariable analyses?

Yes. *Multivariable Analysis: A Practical Guide for Clinicians* is precisely the reference that will lead your way. In fact, Dr. Mitchell Katz has asked and answered all of your questions for you!

Why should I do multivariable analysis?
How do I choose which type of multivariable to use?
How many subjects do I need to do multivariable analysis?
Does it matter if my independent variables are related to each other?
How can I validate my models?

Answers and detailed explanations to these questions and more are found in this book. Also, it is loaded with useful tips, summary charts, figures, and references. Instead of following one or two data sets, it uses examples from the medical literature to demonstrate the many different ways of applying and performing multivariable analysis.

If you are a medical student, resident, or clinician, *Multivariable Analysis: A Practical Guide for Clinicians* will prove an indispensable guide through the confusing terrain of statistical analysis.

Dr. Mitchell H. Katz is Associate Clinical Professor of Medicine, Epidemiology, and Biostatistics at the University of California, San Francisco, as well as an attending physician in San Francisco General Hospital's AIDS and Oncology Division. He is the Director of the San Francisco Department of Public Health.

Multivariable Analysis

A Practical Guide for Clinicians

MITCHELL H. KATZ

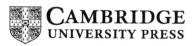

CAMBRIDGE
UNIVERSITY PRESS

PUBLISHED BY THE PRESS SYNDICATE OF THE UNIVERSITY OF CAMBRIDGE
The Pitt Building, Trumpington Street, Cambridge, United Kingdom

CAMBRIDGE UNIVERSITY PRESS
The Edinburgh Building, Cambridge CB2 2RU, UK
40 West 20th Street, New York, NY 10011-4211, USA
10 Stamford Road, Oakleigh, VIC 3166, Australia
Ruiz de Alarcón 13, 28014 Madrid, Spain
Dock House, The Waterfront, Cape Town 8001, South Africa

http://www.cambridge.org

First published 1999
Reprinted 2000, 2001

Printed in the United States of America

Typeset in Stone Serif 9.5/13pt. and Avenir in LaTeX 2_ε [TB]

*A catalog record for this book is available from
the British Library*

Library of Congress Cataloging-in-Publication Data
Katz, Mitchell H.
    Multivariable analysis : a practical guide for clinicians /
Mitchell H. Katz.
        p.   cm.
      1. Medicine – Research – Statistical methods.   2. Multivariate
analysis.   3. Biometry.   4. Medical statistics.   I. Title.
    R853.S7K38   1999
    610′. 7′27 – dc21   98–39350
                                                                        CIP

ISBN 0 521 59301 8 hardback
ISBN 0 521 59693 9 paperback

Contents

CONTENTS

Preface

I decided to write a statistics book because, as both a researcher and a teacher of research, I felt frustrated at the absence of an easy to read text on multivariable analysis. Most existing texts are too difficult for the beginning researcher. Although there are some basic biostatistics books that can be understood by nonstatisticians, most of these do not cover multivariable analysis. I wanted to write the kind of book that I was looking for when I first began using multivariable models, the kind of book that I could give clinical researchers performing their first research project that requires multivariable analysis. I hope that this is that book.

The book is designed to be easy to follow. No mathematics is required. There are no derivations and few formulas of any kind. Instead I have focused on *conceptual* explanations of what the models are doing and how to interpret the output. I have used a question and answer format to ask and answer the most practical questions. My experience with most statistical books is that they do not answer the basic questions, such as, "What does it mean if the coefficient has a negative sign?" (see Section 9.3). I have included many summary tables, rules of thumb, and analysis tips throughout the book. My hope is that after reading it, you will be able to conduct and interpret most multivariable analyses without the help of a biostatistician. For sophisticated analyses that require the help of a biostatistician, I have tried to provide enough information to explain what needs to be done, even if you end up needing some help to do it.

I have included a large number of examples from the medical literature to illustrate the major points of the book. I chose this strategy, rather than relying on one or two data sets, for several reasons. Most importantly, I wanted readers to feel the excitement that I feel about the numerous and diverse applications of multivariable analysis. Related to this, I wanted researchers to appreciate that there are a number of different ways to accomplish the same goal. Researchers who feel certain that one method of analysis is always better than another (e.g., stepwise regression should always be done by backward elimination rather than forward selection) may object to this approach. There are, of course, reasons for favoring one acceptable method over another. If the effect is true and strong, you will get similar answers with different methods. Indeed, if the effect of interest is present when you do the analysis in one way, but invisible when you perform the analysis in a different, albeit acceptable way, it is likely spurious or very weak.

No textbook is written in a vacuum. I feel a tremendous debt to the writers of several biostatistics books from whom I have learned a great deal. In particular, S. Glantz's *Primer of Biostatistics* (4th ed., McGraw-Hill, 1997) was my first biostatistics book (then in its first edition!), and it would serve as an excellent prerequisite to this book. S. Glantz and B. Slinker's *Primer of Applied Regression and Analysis of Variance* (McGraw-Hill, 1990) is an excellent second book of biostatistics. It covers some of the same material as this text but provides a more detailed explanation of analysis of variance. D. W. Hosmer and S. Lemeshow's *Applied Logistic Regression* (Wiley, 1989) is a classic text and goes into greater depth on this technique than this book. A. Feinstein's *Multivariable Analysis* (Yale University Press, 1996) covers much of the same ground but takes a different and complementary approach. Other important texts are referenced in footnotes.

My greatest debts are to my teachers, students, and colleagues. Chaya Piotrkowski taught me how to use software packages, as well as how to keypunch computer cards. (Oh, the joys that you have missed if you have recently come of age with computers!) Daniel Singer got me started in clinical research and provided my introduction to logistic regression. Warren Browner, Steven Cummings, Deborah Grady, Stephen Hulley, and Thomas Newman taught me how to think about and teach biostatistics. Walter Hauck helped me struggle through proportional hazards analysis. Former students Alan Chan, Karla Kerlikowske, and Anthony So challenged me to teach them these techniques, and I learned them better in the process. Several years of students in the University of California, San Francisco, Clinical Research Program have contributed to this book through their insightful questions and observations. At the San Francisco Department of Public Health I have been extremely fortunate to work with smart, creative clinical researchers, including Tomas Aragon, Susan Buchbinder,

Jan Gurley, Nancy Hessol, Willi McFarland, Rani Marx, and Sandy Schwarcz. They have taught me much. I owe a special thank you to Eric Vittinghoff, who carefully reviewed the manuscript and recommended a number of important changes. If any errors crept in despite his review, I am only to blame. My friend and colleague, Walter Mebane, has patiently instructed me on statistics and computers since our university days. My friends, David French and Perri Klass, have cheered me on throughout the process.

The figures in the book were artfully drawn by Ward Ruth of Biomed Art Associates. In completing the book, I appreciate the support of my editor Jo-Ann Strangis and the staff at Cambridge University Press.

San Francisco, California
October 1998

1

Introduction

1.1 Why should I do multivariable analysis?

We live in a multivariable world. Most events, whether medical, political, social, or personal, have multiple causes. And these causes are related to one another. Multivariable analysis[1] is a statistical tool for determining the relative contributions of different causes to a single event or outcome.

    Clinical researchers, in particular, need multivariable analysis because most diseases have multiple causes and prognosis is usually determined by a large number of factors. Even for those infectious diseases that are known to be caused by a single pathogen, a number of factors affect whether an exposed individual becomes ill, including the characteristics of the pathogen (e.g., virulence of strain), the route of exposure (e.g., respiratory route), the intensity of exposure (e.g., size of innoculum), and the host response (e.g., immunologic defense).

    Multivariable analysis allows us to sort out the multifaceted nature of risk factors and their relative contribution to outcome. For example, observational epidemiology has taught us that there are a number of risk factors associated with premature mortality, notably smoking, a sedentary lifestyle, obesity, elevated cholesterol, and hypertension. Note that I did not say that these factors *cause* premature mortality. Statistics alone cannot prove that a relationship between a risk factor

> ⫸ **DEFINITION**
>
> *Multivariable analysis* is a tool for determining the relative contributions of different causes to a single event.

---

[1] The terms "multivariate analysis" and "multivariable analysis" are often used interchangeably. In the strict sense, multivariate analysis refers to simultaneously predicting multiple outcomes. Since this book deals with techniques that use multiple variables to predict a single outcome, I prefer the more general term multivariable analysis.

and an outcome are causal.[2] Causality is established on the basis of biological plausibility and rigorous study designs, such as randomized controlled trials, which eliminate sources of potential bias.

Identification of risk factors of premature mortality through observational studies has been particularly important because you cannot randomize people to many of the conditions that cause premature mortality, such as smoking, sedentary lifestyle, or obesity. And yet these conditions tend to occur together; that is, people who smoke tend to exercise less and be more likely to be obese. How does multivariable analysis separate the *independent* contribution of each of these factors? Let's consider the case of exercise. Numerous studies have shown that persons who exercise live longer than persons with sedentary lifestyles. But if the only reason that persons who exercise live longer is that they are less likely to smoke and more likely to eat low fat meals leading to lower cholesterol, then initiating an exercising routine would not change a person's life expectancy.

The Aerobics Center Longitudinal Study tackled this important question.[3] They evaluated the relationship between exercise and mortality in 25,341 men and 7,080 women. All participants had a baseline examination between 1970 and 1989. The examination included a physical examination, laboratory tests, and a treadmill evaluation to assess physical fitness. Participants were followed for an average of 8.4 years for the men and 7.5 years for the women.

Table 1.1 compares the characteristics of survivors to persons who had died during the follow-up. You can see that there are a number of significant differences between survivors and decedents among men and women. Specifically, survivors were younger, had lower blood pressure, lower cholesterol, were less likely to smoke, and were more physically fit (based on the length of time they stayed on the treadmill and their level of effort).

Although the results are interesting, Table 1.1 does not answer our basic question: Does being physically fit independently increase

---

[2] Throughout the text I use the terms "associated with" and "related to" interchangeably. Similarly, I use the terms "risk factor" and "independent variable," and the terms "outcome" and "dependent variable," interchangeably. Although many use the term "predicts" to refer to the association between an independent variable and an outcome, the term implies causality and I prefer to reserve it for when we are determining how well a model predicts the outcome of individual subjects (Section 9.2C).

[3] Blair, S.N., Kampert, J.B., Kohl, H.W., et al. "Influences of cardiorespiratory fitness and other precursors on cardiovascular disease and all-cause mortality in men and women." *JAMA* 1996;276:205–10.

INTRODUCTION

TABLE 1.1

Baseline characteristics of survivors and decedents, Aerobics Center Longitudinal Study.

Characteristics	Men		Women	
	Survivors (n = 24,740)	Decedents (n = 601)	Survivors (n = 6,991)	Decedents (n = 89)
Age, y (SD)	42.7 (9.7)	52.1 (11.4)	42.6 (10.9)	53.3 (11.2)
Body mass index, kg/m^2 (SD)	26.0 (3.6)	26.3 (3.5)	22.6 (3.9)	23.7 (4.5)
Systolic blood pressure, mm Hg (SD)	121.1 (13.5)	130.4 (19.1)	112.6 (14.8)	122.6 (17.3)
Total cholesterol, mg/dL (SD)	213.1 (40.6)	228.9 (45.4)	202.7 (40.5)	228.2 (40.8)
Fasting glucose, mg/dL (SD)	100.4 (16.3)	108.1 (32.0)	94.4 (14.5)	99.9 (25.0)
Fitness, %				
Low	20.1	41.6	18.8	44.9
Moderate	42.0	39.1	40.6	33.7
High	37.9	19.3	40.6	21.3
Current or recent smoker, %	26.3	36.9	18.5	30.3
Family history of coronary heart disease, %	25.4	33.8	25.2	27.0
Abnormal electrocardiogram, %	6.9	26.3	4.8	18.0
Chronic illness, %	18.4	40.3	13.4	20.2

Adapted with permission from Blair, S.N., et al. "Influences of cardiorespiratory fitness and other precursors on cardiovascular disease and all-cause mortality in men and women." *JAMA* 1996;276:205–10. Copyright 1996, American Medical Association. Additional data provided by authors.

longevity? It doesn't answer the question because whereas the high-fitness group was less likely to die during the study period, those who were physically fit may just have been younger, been less likely to smoke, or had lower blood pressure.

To determine whether exercise is independently associated with mortality, the authors performed proportional hazards analysis, a type of multivariable analysis. The results are shown in Table 1.2. If you compare the number of deaths per thousand person-years in men, you can see that there were more deaths in the low-fitness group (38.1)

TABLE 1.2
Multivariable analysis of risk factors for all-cause mortality, Aerobics Center Longitudinal Study.

Independent variable	Men		Women	
	Deaths per 10,000 person-years	Adjusted relative risk (95% CI)	Deaths per 10,000 person-years	Adjusted relative risk (95% CI)
Fitness				
Low	38.1	1.52 (1.28–1.82)	27.8	2.10 (1.36–3.26)
Moderate/High	25.0	1.0 (ref.)	13.2	1.0 (ref.)
Smoking Status				
Current or recent smoker	39.4	1.65 (1.39–1.97)	27.8	1.99 (1.25–3.17)
Past or never smoked	23.9	1.0 (ref.)	14.0	1.0 (ref.)
Systolic blood pressure				
$\geq$140 mm Hg	35.6	1.30 (1.08–1.58)	13.0	0.76 (0.41–1.40)
<140 mm Hg	27.3	1.0 (ref.)	17.1	1.0 (ref.)
Cholesterol				
$\geq$240 mg/dL	35.1	1.34 (1.13–1.59)	18.0	1.09 (0.68–1.74)
<240 mg/dL	26.1	1.0 (ref.)	16.6	1.0 (ref.)
Family history of coronary heart disease				
Yes	29.9	1.07 (0.90–1.29)	12.8	0.70 (0.43–1.16)
No	27.8	1.0 (ref.)	18.2	1.0 (ref.)
Body mass index				
$\geq$27 kg/m^2	28.8	1.02 (0.86–1.22)	15.9	0.94 (0.52–1.69)
<27 kg/m^2	28.2	1.0 (ref.)	16.9	1.0 (ref.)
Fasting glucose				
$\geq$120 mg/dL	34.4	1.24 (0.98–1.56)	29.6	1.79 (0.80–4.00)
<120 mg/dL	27.9	1.0 (ref.)	16.5	1.0 (ref.)
Abnormal electrocardiogram				
Yes	44.4	1.64 (1.34–2.01)	25.3	1.55 (0.87–2.77)
No	27.1	1.0 (ref.)	16.3	1.0 (ref.)
Chronic illness				
Yes	41.2	1.63 (1.37–1.95)	17.5	1.05 (0.61–1.82)
No	25.3	1.0 (ref.)	16.7	1.0 (ref.)

Adapted with permission from Blair, S.N., et al. "Influences of cardiorespiratory fitness and other precursors on cardiovascular disease and all-cause mortality in men and women." *JAMA* 1996;276:205–10. Copyright 1996, American Medical Association. Additional data provided by authors.

TABLE 1.3
Stratified analysis of smoking and fitness on all-cause mortality among men, Aerobics Center Longitudinal Study.

	Deaths per 10,000 person-years	Stratum-specific relative risk (95% CI)
Smokers		
Low fitness	48.0	1.63 (1.26–2.13)
Moderate/high fitness	29.4	1.0 (ref.)
Nonsmokers		
Low fitness	44.0	2.19 (1.77–2.70)
Moderate/high fitness	20.1	1.0 (ref.)

Data supplied by Aerobics Center Longitudinal Study.

than in the moderate/high-fitness group (25.0). This difference is reflected in the elevated relative risk for lower fitness (38.1/25.0 = 1.52). These results are adjusted for all of the other variables listed in the table. This means that low fitness is associated with higher mortality independent of the effects of other known risk factors for mortality, such as smoking, elevated blood pressure, cholesterol, and family history. A similar pattern is seen for women.

Was there any way to answer this question without multivariable analysis? One could have performed stratified analysis. Stratified analysis assesses the effect of a risk factor on outcome while holding another variable constant. So, for example, we could compare physically fit to unfit persons separately among smokers and nonsmokers. This would allow us to calculate a relative risk for the impact of fitness on mortality, independent of smoking. This analysis is shown in Table 1.3.

Unlike the multivariable analysis in Table 1.2, the analyses in Table 1.3 are bivariate.[4] We see that the mortality rate is greater among those at low fitness compared to those at moderate/high fitness both among smokers (48.0 vs. 29.4) and among nonsmokers (44.0 vs. 20.1).

> **▶ DEFINITION**
>
> *Stratified analysis* assesses the effect of a risk factor on outcome while holding another variable constant.

---

[4] Some researchers use the term "univariate" to describe the association between two variables. I think it is more informative to restrict the term univariate to analyses of a single variable (e.g., mean, median), while using the term "bivariate" to refer to the association between two variables.

This stratified analysis shows that the effect of fitness is independent of smoking status.

But what about all of the other variables that might affect the relationship between fitness and longevity? You could certainly stratify for each one individually, proving that the effect of fitness on longevity is independent not only of smoking status, but also independent of elevated cholesterol, elevated blood pressure, and so on. However, this would only prove that the relationship is independent of these variables taken singly. To stratify by two variables (smoking and cholesterol), you would have to assess the relationship between fitness and mortality in four groups (smokers with high cholesterol; smokers with low cholesterol; nonsmokers with high cholesterol; nonsmokers with low cholesterol). To stratify by three variables (smoking status, cholesterol level, and elevated blood pressure (yes/no)), you would have to assess the relationship between fitness and mortality in eight groups; add elevated glucose (yes/no) and you would have 16 groups; add age (in six decades) and you would have 96 groups; and we haven't even yet taken into account all of the variables in Table 1.1 that are associated with mortality.

With each stratification variable you add, you increase the number of subgroups for which you have to individually assess whether the relationship between fitness and mortality holds. Besides producing mountains of printouts, and requiring a book (rather than a journal article) to report your results, you would likely have an insufficient sample size in some of these subgroups, even if you started with a large sample size. For example, in the Aerobics Center Longitudinal Study there were 25,341 men but only 601 deaths. With 96 subgroups, assuming uniform distributions, you would expect only about 6 deaths per subgroup. But, in reality you wouldn't have uniform distributions. Some samples would be very small, and some would have no outcomes at all.

Multivariable analysis overcomes this limitation. It allows you to simultaneously assess the impact of multiple independent variables on outcome. But there is (always) a cost: The model makes certain assumptions about the nature of the data. These assumptions are sometimes hard to verify. We will take up these issues in Chapters 5, 6, 7, and 10.

1.2 What are confounders and how does multivariable analysis help me to deal with them?

The ability of multivariable analysis to *simultaneously* assess the independent contribution of a number of risk factors to outcome is

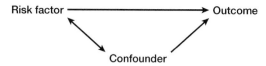

Figure 1.1. Relationships among risk factor, confounder, and outcome.

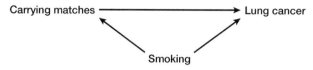

Figure 1.2. Relationships among carrying matches, smoking, and lung cancer.

particularly important when you have confounding. Confounding occurs when the apparent association between a risk factor and an outcome is affected by the relationship of a third variable to the risk factor and the outcome; the third variable is called a confounder.

For a variable to be a confounder, the variable must be associated with the risk factor and causally related to the outcome (Figure 1.1).

A classically taught example of confounding is the relationship between carrying matches and developing lung cancer (Figure 1.2). Persons who carry matches have a greater chance of developing lung cancer; the confounder is smoking. This example is often used to illustrate confounding because it is easy to grasp that carrying matches cannot possibly cause lung cancer.

Stratified analysis can be used to assess and eliminate confounding. If you stratify by smoking status you will find that carrying matches is not associated with lung cancer. That is, there will be no relationship between carrying matches and lung cancer when you look separately among smokers and nonsmokers. The statistical evidence of confounding is the difference between the unstratified and the stratified analysis. In the unstratified analysis the chi-square test would be significant and the odds ratio for the impact of matches on lung cancer would be significantly greater than one. In the two stratified analyses (smokers and nonsmokers), carrying matches would not be significantly associated with lung cancer; the odds ratio would be one in both strata. This differs from the example of stratified analysis in Table 1.3 where exercise was significantly associated with mortality for both smokers and nonsmokers.

Most clinical examples of confounding are more subtle and harder to diagnose than the case of matches and lung cancer. Let's look at the

> **▐▶ DEFINITION**
>
> A *confounder* is associated with the risk factor and causally related to the outcome.

TABLE 1.4

Bivariate association between smoking status and risk of death.

Bivariate	Nonsmokers	Former smokers	Recent quitters	Persistent smokers
Relative risk of death	1.0 (ref.)	1.08 (.92–1.26)	.56 (.40–.77)	.74 (.59–.94)

Adapted from Hasdai, D., et al. "Effect of smoking status on the long-term outcome after successful percutaneous coronary revascularization." *N. Engl. J. Med.* 1997;336:755–61.

relationship between smoking and prognosis in patients with coronary artery disease following angioplasty (the opening of clogged coronary vessels with the use of a wire and a balloon).

Everyone knows (although the cigarette companies long claimed ignorance) that smoking increases the risk of death. Countless studies including the Aerobics Center Longitudinal Study (Table 1.2) have demonstrated that smoking is associated with increased mortality. How then can we explain the results of Hasdai and colleagues?[5] They followed 5,437 patients with coronary artery disease who had angioplasty. They divided their sample into nonsmokers, former smokers (quit at least six months before procedure), quitters (quit immediately following the procedure), and persistent smokers. The relative risk of death with the 95% confidence intervals are shown in Table 1.4.

How can the risk of death be lower among persons who persistently smoke than those who never smoked? In the case of recent quitters, you would expect their risk of death to return toward normal only after years of not smoking – and even then you wouldn't actually expect quitters to have a lower risk of death.

Before you assume that there is something wrong with this study, several other studies have found a similar relationship between smoking and better prognosis among patients with coronary artery disease after thrombolytic therapy. This effect has been named the "smoker's

[5] Hasdai, D., Garratt, K.N., Grill, D.E., Lerman, A., Homes, D.R. "Effect of smoking status on the long-term outcome after successful percutaneous coronary revascularization." *N. Engl. J. Med.* 1997;336:755–61.

TABLE 1.5

Association between demographic and clinical factors and smoking status.

	Nonsmokers	Former smokers	Recent quitters	Persistent smokers
Age, year $\pm$ SD	67 ± 11	65 ± 10	56 ± 10	55 ± 11
Duration of angina, month $\pm$ SD	41 ± 66	51 ± 72	21 ± 46	29 ± 55
Diabetes, %	21%	18%	8%	10%
Hypertension, %	54%	48%	38%	39%
Extent of coronary artery disease, %				
One vessel	50%	51%	57%	55%
Two vessels	36%	36%	34%	36%
Three vessels	14%	13%	10%	9%

Adapted from Hasdai, D., et al. "Effect of smoking status on the long-term outcome after successful percutaneous coronary revascularization." *N. Engl. J. Med.* 1997;336:755–61.

paradox."[6] What is behind the paradox? Look at Table 1.5. As you can see, compared to nonsmokers and former smokers, quitters and persistent smokers are younger, have had angina for a shorter period of time, are less likely to have diabetes and hypertension, and have less severe coronary artery disease (i.e., more one-vessel disease and less three-vessel disease). Given this, it is not so surprising that the recent quitters and persistent smokers have a lower risk of death than nonsmokers and former smokers: They are younger and have fewer underlying medical problems than the nonsmokers and former smokers.

Compare the bivariate (unadjusted) risk of death to the multivariable risk of death (Table 1.6). Note that in the multivariable analysis the researchers adjusted for those differences, such as age and duration of angina, that existed among the four groups.

With statistical adjustment for the baseline differences between the groups, the quitters and persistent smokers have a significantly

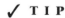

✓ **TIP**

Multivariable analysis is preferable to stratified analysis when you have multiple confounders.

[6] Barbash, G.I., Reiner, J., White, H.D., et al. "Evaluation of paradoxical beneficial effects of smoking in patients receiving thrombolytic therapy for acute myocardial infarction: Mechanisms of the 'smoker's paradox' from the GUSTO-I trial, with angiographic insights." *J. Am. Coll. Cardiol.* 1995;26:1222–9.

TABLE 1.6
Comparison of bivariate and multivariable association between smoking status and risk of death.

	Nonsmokers	Former smokers	Recent quitters	Persistent smokers
Relative risk of death				
Bivariate	1.0 (ref.)	1.08 (.92–1.26)	.56 (.40–.77)	.74 (.59–.94)
Relative risk of death				
Multivariable	1.0 (ref.)	1.34 (1.14–1.57)	1.21 (.87–1.70)	1.76 (1.37–2.26)

Adapted from Hasdai, D., et al. "Effect of smoking status on the long-term outcome after successful percutaneous coronary revascularization." *N. Engl. J. Med.* 1997;336:755–61.

greater risk of death than nonsmokers – a much more sensible result. (The quitters also have a greater risk of death than the nonsmokers, but the confidence intervals of the relative risk do not exclude one.) The difference between the bivariate and multivariable analysis indicates that confounding is present. The advantage of multivariable analysis over stratified analysis is that it would have been difficult to stratify for age, duration of angina, diabetes, hypertension, and extent of coronary artery disease.

Although the use of multivariable models to adjust for multiple confounders has been a major boon for epidemiology, it is possible to be over zealous in adjusting for potential confounders and thereby adjust away the very effect you are trying to demonstrate. Camargo and colleagues recognized this in their study of the relationship between moderate alcohol consumption and risk of heart attack.[7] Sensibly, they adjusted for age, smoking, exercise, diabetes, and family history of heart attack. However, they did not adjust for blood pressure, body mass index, or hypercholesterolemia. Why not? After all, these factors fit the definition of a confounder, in that they are associated with the risk factor (alcohol consumption) and causally related to the outcome (myocardial infarction). The problem is that alcohol consumption can cause elevations in blood pressure, body mass index, and hypercholesterolemia. Therefore, as illustrated in Figure 1.3, these variables may be

> ⏩ **DEFINITION**
>
> An *intervening variable* is on the causal pathway to your outcome.

---

[7] Camargo, C.A., Stampfer, M.J., Glynn, R.J., et al. "Moderate alcohol consumption and risk for angina pectoris or myocardial infarction in U.S. male physicians." *Ann. Intern. Med.* 1997;126:372–5.

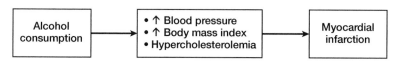

Figure 1.3. Hypothesized pathway by which alcohol consumption may cause myocardial infarction.

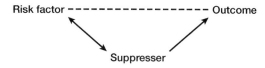

Figure 1.4. Relationships among risk factor, suppresser, and outcome.

on the causal pathway to myocardial infarction and should be thought of as intervening variables rather than as confounders. If you adjust for intervening variables, as if they were confounders, you will adjust away the effect you are trying to demonstrate.

Statistics cannot tell you whether something is a confounder or an intervening variable. Statistically, confounders and intervening variables operate the same. Whether to include a variable in your model because you believe it is a confounder, or exclude it because you believe it is an intervening variable, is a decision you must make based on prior research and biological plausibility.

> ✓ **TIP**
>
> Statistics cannot distinguish between a confounder and an intervening variable.

1.3 What are suppressers and how does multivariable analysis help me to deal with them?

Suppresser variables are a type of confounder. As with confounders, a suppresser is associated with the risk factor and the outcome (Figure 1.4). The difference is that on bivariate analysis there is no effect seen between the risk factor and the outcome. But when you adjust for the suppresser, the relationship between the risk factor and the outcome become significant.

Identifying and adjusting for suppressers can lead to important findings. For example, it was unknown whether taking antiretroviral treatment would prevent HIV seroconversion among health care workers who sustained a needle stick from a patient who was HIV-infected. For several years, health care workers who had an exposure were offered zidovudine treatment, but they were told that there was no efficacy data to support its use. A randomized controlled trial was attempted, but it was disbanded because health care workers did not wish to be randomized.

> ✓ **TIP**
>
> Unlike a typical confounder, when you have a suppresser you won't see any bivariate association between the risk factor and the outcome until you adjust for the suppresser.

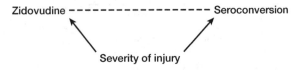

Figure 1.5. Bivariate relationships among zidovudine, severity of injury, and seroconversion.

Since a randomized controlled trial was not possible, a case-control study was performed instead.[8] The cases were health care workers who sustained a needle stick and had seroconverted. The controls were health care workers who sustained a needle stick but had remained HIV-negative. The question was whether the proportion of persons taking zidovudine would be lower in the group who had seroconverted (the cases) than in the group who had not become infected (the controls). The investigators found that the proportion of cases using zidovudine was lower (9 of 33 cases or 27%) than the proportion of controls using zidovudine (247 of 679 controls or 36%), but the difference was not statistically significant (probability $(P) = .35$). Consistent with this nonsignificant trend, the odds ratio shows that zidovudine was protective (0.7), but the 95% confidence intervals were wide and did not exclude one (0.3–1.4).

However, it was known that health care workers who sustained an especially serious exposure (e.g., a deep injury or who stuck themselves with a needle that had visible blood on it) were more likely to choose to take zidovudine than health care workers who had more minor exposures. Also, health care workers who had serious exposures were more likely to seroconvert.

When the researchers adjusted their analysis for severity of injury using multiple logistic regression, zidovudine use was associated with a significantly lower risk of seroconversion (odds ratio $(OR) = 0.2$; 95% confidence interval $(CI) = 0.1$–0.6; $p < 0.01$). Thus, we have an example of a suppresser effect as shown in Figure 1.5. Severity of exposure is associated with zidovudine use and causally related to seroconversion. Zidovudine use is not associated with seroconversion in bivariate analyses but becomes significant when you adjust for severity of injury.

[8] Cardo, D.M., Culver, D.H., Ciesielski, C.A., et al. "A case-control study of HIV seroconversion in health-care workers after percutaneous exposure." *N. Engl. J. Med.* 1997;337:1485–90.

INTRODUCTION

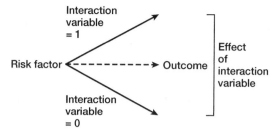

Figure 1.6. Illustration of an interaction effect.

Although this multivariable analysis demonstrated the efficacy of zidovudine on seroconversion by incorporating the suppresser variables, it should be remembered that multivariable analysis cannot adjust for other potential biases in the analysis. For example, the cases and controls for this study were not chosen from the same population, raising the possibility that selection bias may have influenced the results. Nonetheless, on the strength of this study, postexposure prophylaxis with antiretroviral treatment became the standard of care for health care workers who sustained needle sticks from HIV-contaminated needles.

1.4 What are interactions and how does multivariable analysis help me to deal with them?

An interaction occurs when the impact of a risk factor on outcome is changed by the value of a third variable. Interaction is sometimes referred to as effect modification, since the effect of the risk factor on outcome is modified by another variable.

An interaction is illustrated in Figure 1.6. The risk factor's effect on outcome (solid lines) differs depending on the value of the interaction variable (whether it is 1 or 0). The dotted line indicates the relationship without consideration of the interaction effect.

In extreme cases, an interaction may completely reverse the relationship between the risk factor and the outcome. This would occur when the risk factor increased the likelihood of outcome at one value of the interaction variable but decreased the likelihood of outcome at a different value of the interaction variable. More commonly, the effect of the risk factor on the outcome is stronger (or weaker) at certain values of the third variable.

As with confounding, stratification can be used to identify an interaction. By stratifying by the interaction variable, you can observe

> **DEFINITION**
>
> An *interaction* occurs when the impact of a risk factor on outcome is changed by the value of a third variable.

the effect of a risk factor on outcome at the different values of the interaction variable. You can statistically test whether the association between a risk factor and an outcome at different levels of the interaction variable are statistically different from one another using a chi-square test for homogeneity.

However, as with the use of stratification to eliminate confounding, use of stratification to demonstrate interaction has limitations. It is cumbersome to stratify by more than one or two variables; yet you may have multiple interactions in your data. Whereas stratification will accurately quantify the effect of the risk factor on the outcome at different levels of the interaction variable, this analysis will not be adjusted for the other variables in your model (e.g., confounders) that may affect the relationship between risk factor and outcome. Multivariable analysis allows you to include interaction terms and assess them while adjusting for other variables.

For example, Zucker and colleagues evaluated whether specific signs or symptoms of myocardial infarction were different in men than in women presenting to the emergency department with chest pain or other symptoms of acute cardiac ischemia.[9]

In Table 1.7 you can see the association between the independent variables and confirmed diagnoses of acute myocardial infarction. The coefficients and odds ratios are from a multiple logistic regression model. The authors found three significant interactions involving gender: male gender and ST elevation (on electrocardiogram), male gender and congestive heart failure, and male gender and white race.

What do these interactions mean? Let's use the interaction involving male gender and ST elevations as an example (I have put these two variables and their interaction term in bold print). Note that men were more likely than women to have cardiac ischemia ($OR = 1.6$), even after adjusting for other variables associated with ischemia. Similarly, ST elevations were more likely to indicate ischemia ($OR = 8.1$). Given this, you would expect that males with ST elevations would have markedly higher risk of myocardial infarction ($1.6 \times 8.1 = 13.0$) than women ($1.0 \times 8.1 = 8.1$) (the wonderful property of odds ratios that allows you to multiply them this way is explained in Section 10.8).

The multiplication of the odds ratios of gender and ST elevations would lead you to believe that men with ST elevations would have

[9] Zucker, D.R., Griffith, J.L., Beshansky, J.R., Selker, H.P. "Presentations of acute myocardial infarction in men and women." *J. Gen. Intern. Med.* 1997;12:79–87.

TABLE 1.7

Association of independent variables with confirmed diagnosis of acute myocardial infarction based on multiple logistic regression model.

Independent variables	Coefficients	Odds ratio
Male gender	**0.4852**	**1.6**
Age <50	0.1432	1.2
Chest pain	0.8792	2.4
Chief complaint: chest pain	0.4399	1.6
Nausea/vomiting	0.5153	1.7
Congestive heart failure	0.6759	2.0
White race	0.0987	1.1
ST elevation	**2.0948**	**8.1**
ST depression	1.2632	3.5
Q waves	0.5311	1.7
History of diabetes mellitus	0.2781	1.3
History of hypertension	0.2032	1.2
History of angina	−0.2976	0.7
History of peptic ulcers	−0.3210	0.7
Dizziness	−0.4437	0.6
Interactions		
Male gender and congestive heart failure	−0.6899	0.5
Male gender and ST elevation	**−0.5187**	**0.6**
Male gender and white race	0.5206	1.7

Adapted with permission from Zucker, D.R., et al. "Presentation of acute myocardial infarction in men and women." *J. Gen. Intern. Med.* 1997;12:79–87.

significantly higher risk of heart attack than women (13.0 vs. 8.1). In fact, the risk for men and women with ST elevations was similar. This is reflected in the negative coefficient for male gender × ST elevations and the odds ratio of 0.6. If you multiply out the odds ratio for the interaction of male gender with ST elevations, men with ST elevations ($1.6 \times 8.1 \times 0.6 = 7.8$) and women with ST elevations ($1.0 \times 8.1 \times 1.0 = 8.1$) have a similar risk of myocardial infarction.

ST elevations are highly specific for (although not diagnostic of) myocardial infarction. It is not surprising, therefore, that the risks of myocardial infarction are similar in men and women with ST elevations. Had being male made it even worse to have ST elevations the coefficient would have been positive, the odds ratio would have been greater than one, and we would have seen an even greater difference between the risk of heart attack for men and for women in the presence of ST elevations than the difference between 13.0 and 8.1.

Because interaction effects can be difficult to assess and interpret, I will return to this topic in Sections 8.3, 9.9, and 10.8.

INTRODUCTION

2

Common Uses of Multivariable Models

2.1 What are the most common uses of multivariable models in clinical research?

Multivariable models have a variety of uses in clinical research, in both nonrandomized and randomized studies. The four most common uses of multivariable models are to:

A. identify prognostic factors while adjusting for potential confounders,
B. adjust for differences in baseline characteristics,
C. determine prognosis (prognostic models),
D. determine diagnosis (diagnostic models).

These four uses are related, and many studies will use multivariable models for several or all of these purposes. Nonetheless, it is worth thinking about them individually to grasp the power and versatility of these models.

2.1.A Identify prognostic factors while adjusting for potential confounders

As we learn more about certain multifactorial diseases, such as cardiac disease, we identify a larger and larger number of risk factors for the disease. Because many of these variables are associated with one another, stratification becomes an unwieldy technique for eliminating confounding. For example, when Garner and colleagues assessed whether the size of low-density lipoprotein particles affected the incidence of coronary artery disease they adjusted their analysis for those risk factors long known to increase the risk of coronary artery disease, such as smoking, blood pressure, and body mass index.[10] But they also adjusted their model for more recently identified risk factors such as HDL cholesterol, non-HDL cholesterol, and triglycerides. One of the most extensive studies of cardiovascular disease, the Framingham study, which began in 1948, did not even collect data on HDL cholesterol until 1972.[11]

✓ **T I P**

Even when there is no evidence of confounding on bivariate analysis, your peers will expect you to perform multivariable analysis to prove that there is no confounding.

What if you can prove that the potential confounders are not confounders? What if you test all potential confounders and find that none are related to both your risk factor and outcome? Do you still need to use multivariable analysis to adjust for these factors or could you just report the bivariate association between the risk factor and the outcome? Technically, in instances where there are no variables associated with both risk factor and outcome, you would not need to use multivariate analysis.[12] Nonetheless, this has become an academic question. In practice, most clinical researchers use multivariable analysis when there are other factors associated with outcome even if these variables are not actual confounders. The reason is that multivariable analysis has become the standard method for proving that there is no confounding. Thus you will often see instances where the association between the risk factor and the outcome are very similar in the bivariate and multivariable analysis, indicating no confounding. Yet, it is the multivariable result that is cited.

Although multivariable models are excellent tools for adjusting for potential confounders, don't assume that just because you have included a potential confounder in your model you have eliminated any bias due to this confounder. In the real world, no adjustment is perfect. Just as there is error in measurement of your dependent and independent variables, there is error in your confounders. Once you appreciate that your measurement of confounding variables is imperfect, you realize that including a variable in a model cannot completely eliminate confounding. Moreover, the models themselves

[10] Gardner, C.D., Fortmann, S.P., Krauss, R.M. "Association of small low-density lipoprotein particles with the incidence of coronary artery disease in men and women." *JAMA* 1996;276:875–81.

[11] Levy, D., Wilson, P.W.F., Anderson, K.M., Castelli, W.P. "Stratifying the patient at risk from coronary disease: New insights from the Framingham heart study." *Am. Heart. J.* 1990;119:712–17.

[12] It is possible for a variable to change the relationship between a risk factor and outcome even though it is related only to the outcome, but this rarely occurs: See Kahn, H.A., Sempos, C.T. *Statistical Methods in Epidemiology*. Oxford: Oxford University Press, 1989, pp. 85–6.

contain error. Important variables may be omitted, they may be incorrectly specified (Section 5.4), or interactions between the variables may not be appropriately accounted for (Section 10.8). This warning is not meant to be discouraging; rather, it is stated to promote humility about what you can and cannot do with statistical models.

2.1.B   Adjustment for differences in baseline characteristics

Adjustment for differences in baseline characteristics is especially important in nonrandomized (observational) trials. With studies of this type the groups being compared are not equivalent since assignment is not determined by randomization.

Although randomization is the best method of assuring that comparison groups are equal at the start of a study, it is not always feasible to randomize subjects. In instances when expense, logistical, or ethical difficulties preclude randomizing patients, multivariable analysis can be used to statistically approximate equal comparison groups. Of course, multivariable analysis can never adjust for unknown or unmeasured confounders. Only randomization can create groups that are equal with respect to both measured and unmeasured confounders.[13]

Multivariable analysis was used to adjust for known confounders in an important nonrandomized study of right heart catheterization in critically ill patients.[14] This procedure involves inserting a monitoring (Swan–Ganz) catheter directly into the right heart. It began to be widely used in the 1970s without any studies proving its efficacy. Many clinicians felt that the readings enabled them to better monitor and treat their patients. Thus, the practice became the standard of care in certain settings. When some studies found higher rates of death in patients who received right heart catheterization, the validity of the association between right heart catherization and death was questioned because the studies were not randomized. In particular, persons who received right heart catheterization were known to be sicker than persons who did not receive this procedure. This could have confounded

✓ T I P

When randomization is impossible, use multivariable analysis to statistically approximate equal comparison groups.

---

[13] For more on the uses of multivariable analysis for observational studies see: Anderson, S., Auquier, A., Hauck, W.W., Oakes, D., Vanaele, W., Weisberg, H.I. *Statistical Methods for Comparative Studies*. New York: Wiley, 1980; Rosati, R.A., Lee, K.L., Califf, R.M., Pryor, D.B., Harrell, F.E. "Problems and advantages of an observational data base approach to evaluating the effect of therapy on outcome." *Circulation* 1982;65(suppl II):27–32.

[14] Connors, A.F., Speroff, T., Dawson, N.V., et al. "The effectiveness of right heart catheterization in the initial care of critically ill patients." *JAMA* 1996;276:889–97.

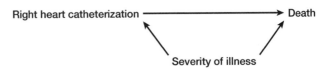

Figure 2.1. Relationships among right heart catheterization, severity of illness, and death.

the results of the observation trials, resulting in persons who received right heart catherization appearing more likely to die because of the catherization when they were, in reality, more likely to die because of their underlying disease. This relationship is illustrated in Figure 2.1.

When a randomized controlled trial was launched to definitively answer the question, the study was terminated because physicians were unwilling to randomize their patients. They believed that right heart catheterization was beneficial; therefore, how could they deny the intervention to their patients?

Connors and colleagues conducted a nonrandomized study of 5,735 critically ill patients. Using multiple logistic regression they developed a propensity score that measured the likelihood of a patient receiving a right heart catheterization. A propensity score is a weighted combination of possible confounders.[15] In this case, the propensity score was based on a large number of potential confounders including age, sex, race, education, type of insurance, type of disease, and several measures of disease severity that affect whether a patient will receive the procedure. When they adjusted for the propensity score for right heart catheterization in a proportional hazards analysis, patients managed with a right heart catheterization had an increased risk of death ($OR = 1.21$; 95% $CI = 1.09-1.25$). The investigators also found that when they matched subjects who did and did not receive right heart catheterization by propensity scores, survival was consistently shorter for those who received right heart catheterization.

Although multivariable analysis can not statistically adjust for unknown or unmeasured confounders, you can attempt to estimate the magnitude of the effect of an unmeasured confounder on your results. For example, Connors and colleagues singly removed from their propensity score variables with the largest effect on the probability of right heart catheterization. They found that removal of any one variable did not change the risk of death. Although this certainly does not

DEFINITION

A *propensity score* is a weighted combination of possible confounders.

[15] Rubin, D.B. "Estimating causal effects from large data sets using propensity scores." *Ann. Intern. Med.* 1997;127:757–63.

COMMON USES OF MULTIVARIABLE MODELS

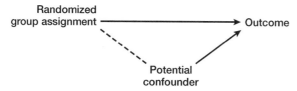

Figure 2.2. Relationships among randomized group assignment, potential confounder, and outcome.

prove that there aren't some unmeasured confounders that alone or in combination are markedly stronger than any of the known confounders in their analysis, it makes it seem less likely.

One ironic aspect of their study is that it may have created enough uncertainty about the use of right heart catherization that a randomized clinical trial will be feasible. Regardless, it is a testimony to the ingenuity of the investigators and the power of multivariable models for adjusting for baseline differences that the accompanying editorial called for the end of right heart catheterization unless a randomized clinical trial could be carried out.[16]

What about randomized controlled trials? Do you need to use multivariable analysis to adjust for baseline differences? Well, ideally, if the randomization has been conducted in a nonbiased way, your comparison groups will be equal with respect to both known and unknown factors. Therefore, there should be no variables associated with the intervention and thus no confounders (Figure 2.2). One can use a simple bivariate test to compare the outcomes for the two groups and determine if the intervention worked.

That being said, it sometimes happens, by chance, that despite randomization one group is significantly different from the other group. For example, Mittelman and colleagues conducted an intervention to delay nursing home placement of patients with Alzheimer disease.[17] They randomized families to a treatment group (counseling and support for caregivers) and a control group. By chance (and bad luck!), the primary caregiver was significantly more likely to be female among the families randomized to the control group than among the families randomized to the treatment group. Moreover, patients of female caregivers were significantly more likely to be placed in a nursing home

[16] Dalen, J.E., Bone, R.C. "Is it time to pull the pulmonary artery catheter?" *JAMA* 1996;276:916–18.

[17] Mittelman, M.S., Ferris, S.H., Shulman, E., Steinberg, G., Levin, B. "A family intervention to delay nursing home placement of patients with Alzheimer disease." *JAMA* 1996;276:1725–31.

(the main outcome of this study). Thus, without adjustment for the gender of the caregiver, the results of the study would have been difficult to interpret. With adjustment for the gender of the caregiver, the authors demonstrated that the treatment was associated with a decrease in nursing home placement.

Although multivariable analysis made the results of the study by Mittelman and colleagues more interpretable, some researchers are opposed to statistically adjusting randomized clinical trials. Remember that the strength of randomized clinical trials is that randomization produces groups that are equal with respect to both known and unknown factors. This is a tremendous advantage because you can never adjust for what you don't know or can't measure. When you statistically adjust a randomized clinical trial, you are adjusting for the known but not the unknown factors. Whether this partial adjustment makes the groups more comparable or not is a matter of debate. What is clear, however, is that statistical adjustment introduces model error. Thus if your randomized clinical trial shows no or only a borderline effect in the bivariate analysis but a statistically significant effect in the multivariate analyses, some readers will be suspicious that the effect is really due to error in the model.

A different and more common use of multivariable analysis in randomized controlled trials is to determine whether other factors besides treatment group are associated with outcome. This use is akin to determining prognostic factors while adjusting for confounders (Section 2.1.A).

2.1.C   Determine prognosis (prognostic models)

How bad is it, Doc? Will the cancer come back? How long do I have to live? These are some of the most difficult questions clinicians face from their patients. Most ethicists and clinicians agree that patients have a right to an honest answer to these questions. While we will never be able to predict the outcome for any one person, multivariable analysis can provide information on the prognosis of a group of patients with a particular set of known prognostic factors.

For example, Schuchter and colleagues developed a prognostic model using logistic regression for estimating 10-year survival in 488 patients with primary melanoma.[18] They prospectively followed

> ✓ **T I P**
>
> The advantage of randomization is that you can never adjust for what you don't know or can't measure.

---

[18] Schuchter, L., Schultz, D.J., Synnestvedt, M., et al. "A prognostic model for predicting a 10-year survival in patients with primary lymphoma." *Ann. Intern. Med.* 1996;125:369–75.

COMMON USES OF MULTIVARIABLE MODELS

patients with primary melanoma. Ten-year survival was 78%. Using multiple logistic regression, they identified four factors associated with survival at ten years (yes/no): age, sex, location (extremity versus axis of body), and lesion thickness. At one extreme, women who were sixty years or younger with a lesion <0.76 mm of thickness on their extremity had an estimated 10-year survival of 99%. At the other extreme, men who were older than sixty with a lesion >3.6 mm of thickness on their trunk had an estimated 10-year survival of only 10%.

This prognostic model illustrates how different survival can be with the same disease but different patient characteristics. Schuchter and colleagues' model correctly predicted outcome in 74% of cases. In other words, if you knew age, sex, location, and lesion thickness, you would correctly predict survival or death at ten years for 74% of the sample.

The cynics among you may say: I can do better than that without any prognostic information. If I predict that all patients will be alive at 10 years, I will be correct in 78% of the cases (10-year survival = 78%). This is true, but you would not have correctly predicted any of the deaths. Methods for judging the success of predictive models are discussed in Section 9.2.

Prognostic models provide valid estimates of risk only for patients with similar characteristics to those in the study population. For example, if the prognostic model is based on a sample of males over the age of fifty, it will not be helpful in predicting the survival of a forty-five year old woman.

Prognostic models work only when there is a known set of risk factors. They are most useful when they include only those variables readily available to a clinician. If the model requires knowing the genetic markers of the cancer, and testing for those markers is not universally available, the model will be of less help.[19]

Even if all these conditions are met, as is the case with the melanoma study, a model will generally not predict outcome prospectively (with new cases) as well as it does retrospectively (with the cases in the data set from which it was developed). Why? Because the models maximize the correct prediction of the outcome based on the values of the independent and dependent variables in the data set. Since data sets are samplings of the population, rather than the population itself,

> ✓ **T I P**
>
> Prognostic models provide valid estimates of risk only for patients with characteristics similar to those in the study population.

---

[19] For an excellent review of using multivariable models to determine prognosis, see Braitman, L.E., Davidoff, F. "Predicting clinical states in individual patients." *Ann. Intern. Med.* 1996;125:406–12.

you will get a slightly different sample (or a very different sample if there was something biased in your sampling) each time you resample the population. Resampling is an important method for validating prognostic models and will be discussed in Section 11.1.

2.1.D Determine diagnosis (diagnostic models)

Multivariable models can identify the best combination of diagnostic information to determine whether a person has a particular disease. The most extensive work on diagnostic algorithms has been done for determining the likelihood of heart attack in patients presenting to emergency departments with chest pain. The reason this question has received so much attention is that the stakes are high. Chest pain is a common presenting symptom in the emergency department. It can be due to something as minor as heartburn or something as serious as a heart attack. Every day, in every emergency department, clinicians decide whom to send home and whom to admit to the coronary care unit. Although coronary care units save lives for patients with acute ischemia, less than half of those receiving this costly intervention actually have ischemia. There is no one test available at the time of emergency department visit that distinguishes those patients who should be admitted from those who could be sent home.

Pozen and colleagues developed a diagnostic model for determining the likelihood that a patient presenting to an emergency department with chest pain had acute ischemia.[20] From 59 different clinical features they identified 7 clinical features that, when used together in a logistic regression model, produced a prediction of ischemia from 0 to 1.0. To determine the usefulness of the model, the researchers gave the results (during the experimental period) to treating physicians before they had to determine whether to admit patients or send them home. During the control period, the physicians were not given the estimates of the probability of acute ischemia. The researchers found that when the physicians were given the information, their decision making improved: In particular, the number of coronary care unit admissions decreased by 30% without any missed cases of ischemia.

So when confronted with a patient with chest pain, do most emergency department physicians whip out their hand-held calculator and

---

[20] Pozen, M.W., D'Agostino, R.B., Selker, H.P., Sytrkowski, P.A., Hood, W.B. "A predictive instrument to improve coronary-care-unit admission practices in acute ischemic heart disease: A prospective multicenter clinical trial." *N. Engl. J. Med.* 1984;310:1273–8.

COMMON USES OF MULTIVARIABLE MODELS

compute the probability of ischemia? Sadly, no. Corey and Merenstein tested the acceptability of this model to physicians by providing a worksheet version of the algorithm in a convenient dispenser in the emergency department, but not requiring the physicians to use them. Physicians used it in only 2.8% of the cases.[21] Low use of well-validated, diagnostic rules by physicians in clinical practice has been noted elsewhere.[22]

The reasons that diagnostic rules are not more widely used are complicated. Physicians, especially in emergency departments, are pressed for time. Pozen's algorithm can be computed in less than 20 seconds, but it requires a preprogrammed hand-held calculator – something most physicians do not carry around with them. Using the worksheet version (if you had one in front of you) it would take you 30–60 seconds to calculate the probability of ischemia. Although this may not seem like a long time, in the emergency department, with many patients in gurneys in front of you, it can seem like an impossibly long task.

Psychological factors also impede the use of diagnostic models by physicians. Medical training has traditionally been akin to apprenticeship. You work with physicians more experienced than yourself until you have enough experience to function on your own. At a certain point, physicians feel that their judgment is accurate (even if studies show that, for some conditions, diagnostic models are more accurate than decisions made by physicians). The physicians in the Corey and Merenstein study complained that they lost confidence in the model when they discovered that two patients with very different characteristics could have the same predicted probability of ischemia. Perhaps, most importantly, as a profession, physicians are not yet comfortable using computer-generated models. But the potential is there. A good diagnostic model can make an intern instantly as good a diagnostician as the head of the department of medicine!

Although developing diagnostic models can be challenging, in one respect they are easier to construct than models designed to identify prognostic factors. In diagnostic settings, causality is unimportant.

> ✓ **T I P**
>
> A good diagnostic algorithm can make an intern as good a diagnostician as the head of the department of medicine!

---

[21] Corey, G.A., Merenstein, J.H. "Applying the acute ischemic heart disease predictive instrument." *J. Fam. Pract.* 1987;25:127–33.

[22] Pearson, S.D., Goldman, L., Garcia, T.B., Cook, E.F., Lee, T.H. "Physician response to a prediction rule for the triage of emergency department patients with chest pain." *J. Gen. Intern. Med.* 1994;9:241–7. Wasson, J.H., Sox, H.C. "Clinical prediction rules: Have they come of age?" *JAMA* 1996;275:641–2. Gehlbach, S.H. "Commentary." *J. Fam. Pract.* 1987;25:132–3.

For example, diagonal ear lobe creases are associated with coronary events even with adjustment for known cardiac risk factors including age, left ventricular ejection fraction, cholesterol level, smoking, diabetes, family history, and obesity.[23] No one believes that ear lobe creases cause coronary events. Looked at from a different point of view, lowering a patient's cholesterol level may decrease the risk of a myocardial infarction, but removing an ear lobe crease with plastic surgery would have no effect on the risk of heart attack. The association of ear lobe creases with coronary events is confounded by some yet to be determined cardiac risk factor.

But a patient's ear crease still provides useful clinical information. This is especially true if you are a paramedic evaluating patients with chest pain in the field and have little other information about them. Thus in constructing diagnostic algorithms, we are interested in variables that together accurately predict outcome regardless of whether the effect is confounded by some other variable. Also, note that because ear lobe creases are not causally related to coronary heart disease, they cannot be considered to be confounders. Therefore, prognostic studies of heart disease do not have to adjust for it as they would adjust for other known risk factors of coronary artery disease.

2.2 How do I choose what type of multivariable analysis to use?

There are many types and ways of performing multivariable analysis. Fortunately, there are only three techniques commonly used by clinical researchers: multiple linear regression, multiple logistic regression, and proportional hazards analysis. The type of multivariable analysis you will use depends primarily on the nature of your outcome variables, your dependent variables, and the hypothesized relationship between your dependent variables and your outcome variable. These issues are discussed in the next three chapters.

---

[23] Elliott, W.J., Powell, L.H. "Diagonal earlobe creases and prognosis in patients with suspected coronary artery disease." *Am. J. Med.* 1996;100:205–11.

COMMON USES OF MULTIVARIABLE MODELS

3

Outcome Variables in Multivariable Analysis

3.1 How does the nature of my outcome variable influence my choice of which type of multivariable analysis to do?

As shown in Table 3.1, the choice of multivariable analysis depends primarily on the type of outcome variable that you have. With an interval variable (also called continuous) each unit (interval) of change on the scale has an equal (numerically) quantifiable value. Examples of interval variables are blood pressure, body weight, and temperature. In these examples, a one unit change at any point on the scale is equal to a millimeter of mercury, a pound (or kilogram), or a degree, respectively.

    A dichotomous variable (the simplest kind of categorical variable) has two discrete values (categories) at a discrete point in time, for example, alive or dead; development of cancer: yes or no. Time to occurrence of a dichotomous event refers to events, such as death or development of cancer, that occur over a period of time (e.g., five years).

3.2 What should I do if my outcome variable is ordinal or nominal?

An ordinal variable has multiple categories that can be ordered. An example of an ordinal variable is the New York Heart Association's functional classification of cardiac function. There are four levels of the scale. Although the four levels can be ordered, there is not a numerically quantifiable difference between level 1 (no limit in physical activity) and level 2 (slight limitation in physical activity). The difference between level 1 and 2 is not equal to the difference between level

TABLE 3.1
Type of outcome variable determines choice of multivariable analysis.

Type of outcome	Example of outcome variable	Type of multivariable analysis
Interval	Blood pressure, weight, temperature	Multiple linear regression
Dichotomous	Death, cancer, intensive care unit admission	Multiple logistic regression
Time to occurrence of a dichotomous event	Time to death, time to cancer	Proportional hazards analysis

3 (marked limitation of physical activity) and level 4 (inability to carry on any physical activity without discomfort).

A nominal variable is a categorical variable with multiple categories that cannot be ordered. An example of a nominal variable is cause of death: cancer, heart disease, infection, or other. Unlike an ordinal variable, you cannot numerically order cause of death.

As you can tell by looking at Table 3.1, ordinal or nominal outcomes are not usually used with the three multivariable models discussed in this book. Nonetheless, there are options available for incorporating these variables in a multivariable analysis.

One option for ordinal and nominal variables is to convert them to a dichotomous outcome. For example, New York Heart Association classification is often grouped as level I and II (mild shortness of breath) or level III and IV (severe shortness of breath). Similarly, cause of death can be cancer: yes or no. Obviously, such groupings result in loss of information.

Alternatively, the data can be analyzed using an adaptation of logistic regression. Ordinal outcomes can be analyzed using proportional odds logistic regression and nominal outcomes can be analyzed using polytomous logistic regression. Because these techniques are not commonly used in medical research, they will not be described here, but readers can obtain more information about these methods from

▸ DEFINITION

A *nominal* variable is a categorical variable with multiple categories that cannot be ordered.

OUTCOME VARIABLES IN MULTIVARIABLE ANALYSIS

other sources.[24] Another technique available for nominal outcomes is discriminant function analysis, which has both similarities to and differences from the three major methods described here.[25]

While I have drawn a distinction between interval and ordinal variables, in practice, there is a gray area. Clinical researchers, especially those interested in the behavioral sciences, often use multiple linear regression to analyze outcome variables that do not strictly fit the definition of an interval variable but function like one. Examples include patient satisfaction, patient self-rated health perception, and level of pain or distress. These variables are typically derived by having respondents rate their degree of satisfaction, sense of health, or level of pain on an arbitrary numeric scale of 1 to 4, 1 to 5, or 1 to 100. The scale may include cues such as 1 = excellent, 2 = very good, 3 = fair, and 4 = poor or 1 = strongly agree, 2 = agree, 3 = no opinion, 4 = disagree, 5 = strongly disagree. These scales are not truly interval because the interval between excellent and very good is not necessarily the same size as the interval between fair and poor. Nonetheless, when these variables are used as dependent variables in multiple linear regression they are likely to work fine as long as their relationships with the independent variables fulfill the assumptions of multiple linear regression (Sections 5.1–5.4).

3.3 What are the advantages of using time to occurrence of a dichotomous event instead of the simpler cumulative outcome of a dichotomous event at a point in time?

With a cross-sectional study and a dichotomous outcome you would normally use multiple logistic regression. There would be no possibility of using proportional hazards analysis to evaluate time to a dichotomous outcome because in a cross-sectional study the independent variables and the outcome are measured at the same time.

However, in longitudinal studies, outcomes occur after the measurement of your independent variables. Assuming a dichotomous

✓ **TIP**

Clinical medicine consists more of treatments than of cures.

---

[24] See Scott, S.C., Goldberg, M.S., Mayo, N.E. "Statistical assessment of ordinal outcomes in comparative studies." *J. Clin. Epidemiol.* 1997;50:45–55. Menard, S. *Applied Logistic Regression Analysis*. Thousand Oaks, CA: Sage Publications, 1995, pp. 80–90.

[25] See Feinstein, A.R. *Multivariable Analysis: An Introduction*. New Haven: Yale University Press, 1996, pp. 431–74.

outcome, you have two choices of how to analyze the data. You can use the simpler cumulative outcome at a particular point in time, as in: the proportion of the subjects who suffered a heart attack within three years. Alternatively, you can use time to heart attack.

Given that cumulative outcome at a point of time is simpler, why do so many published clinical trials use time to outcome? One important reason is that clinical medicine consists more of treatments than of cures. Given this, what matters is how soon the disease occurs, or how long survival is increased.

Figure 3.1 illustrates this principle. We see two survival curves, corresponding to a treatment group and a no treatment group. At two years the same proportion of patients has died (95%). Yet, the time to death is quite different for the two groups. The patients in the treatment group are dying at a slower rate. At one year, 48% of the patients in the no treatment group have died whereas only 5% of those in the treatment group have died.

✓ **T I P**

Time to occurrence models allow inclusion of subjects with differing lengths of follow-up.

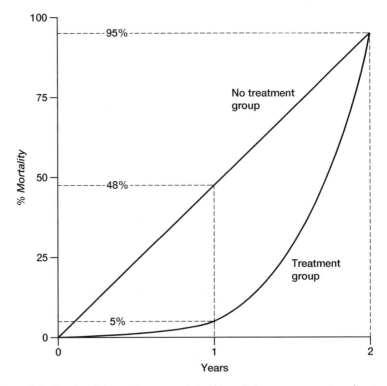

Figure 3.1. Graphs of % mortality versus time. Although the same proportion of patients in both groups are dead at two years, the patients in the treatment group are dying more slowly.

A second reason for preferring time to occurrence models is that they allow you to include in your analysis subjects with differing lengths of follow-up. Differing lengths of follow-up occur in longitudinal studies for many reasons, including study dropouts, study withdrawals, and accrual of study subjects over time. If you use the simpler cumulative outcome of heart attack at three years, and you have a subject who dropped out of your study at two and a half years, you would have to omit the subject from the analysis. With time to occurrence models, this subject could contribute two and a half years of event-free time.

The method for incorporating subjects with variable lengths of follow-up is referred to as censoring. Censoring gives you greater statistical power than you would have if you excluded subjects who did not complete your study. The method is discussed in detail in Sections 7.3–7.5.

One may reasonably ask, especially in these cost-conscious times, how important is an increase in survival of a few months if the ultimate prognosis is the same. The answer to this question is more philosophical than statistical. In general, time to outcome matters more for serious outcomes than for minor ones. Patients with life-threatening diseases value additional time, whether of days or months, especially if it will allow them to see a child graduate from college or watch a grandchild take her first steps.

At the other extreme, for minor outcomes, increased time may not be clinically meaningful. For example, studies have shown that children with chicken pox treated with acyclovir have one day less fever and experience a decrease in the number of chicken pox lesions one day sooner than those given placebo.[26] If the investigators had used symptoms at seven days as the outcome of their study they would have found no effect for acyclovir, because treated or untreated, immunocompetent children with chicken pox are almost invariably well at seven days. Is it worth the expense of acyclovir for one day less of symptoms? Is it worth the trouble (those of you who have attempted to give a toddler a medicine four times a day know what I mean)? Clearly, this is not a statistical question. In practice, although the differences focusing on time to outcome with acyclovir are statistically significant, most pediatricians do not prescribe it for immunocompetent children.

> ⏩ **DEFINITION**
>
> *Censoring* is a method for incorporating subjects with differing lengths of follow-up.

> ✓ **T I P**
>
> Time to outcome matters more for serious outcomes than for minor ones.

---

[26] Balfour, H.H., Kelly, J.M., Suarez, C.S., et al. "Acyclovir treatment of varicella in otherwise healthy children." *J. Pediatr.* 1990;116:633–99.

At times, small improvements in the time to outcome may spur scientific progress, even if there is minimal benefit to individual patients. Most medical advances are incremental. Proving that a particular strategy increases survival, if only marginally, may provide a valuable lead to a better treatment.

In summary, time to outcome is a more sensitive measure than cumulative outcome at a particular point in time. It also allows inclusion of subjects with unequal lengths of follow-up. If you have relatively few outcomes, length of follow-up is relatively short, and few subjects are lost to follow-up, then logistic regression and proportional hazards analysis will provide similar results.[27] This was illustrated in a study of mortality among patients who had coronary angiography and were judged to need coronary revascularization.[28] Of 671 patients, 70 (10.4%) were known to have died, the median follow-up was 797 days, and mortality data were available for all subjects. Multiple logistic regression, adjusted for a number of potential confounders, showed that the odds of death at one year were significantly lower among patients who received coronary revascularization ($OR = 0.49$; 95% $CI = 0.30$–0.84) compared to those who did not receive it. A proportional hazards analysis, which also adjusted for confounders, found that revascularization significantly reduced the risk of death (relative hazard (RH) = 0.59; 95% $CI = 0.36$–$.97$).

[27] Green, M.S., Symons, M.J. "A comparison of the logistic risk function and the proportional hazards model in prospective epidemiologic studies." *J. Chron. Dis.* 1983;36:715–24.

[28] Kravitz, R.L., Laouri, M., Kahan, J.P., et al. "Validity of criteria used for detecting under use of coronary revascularization." *JAMA* 1995;274:632–8.

OUTCOME VARIABLES IN MULTIVARIABLE ANALYSIS

4

Independent Variables in Multivariable Analysis

4.1 What kind of independent variables can I use with multivariable analyses?

Interval and dichotomous independent variables can be used in all three types of multivariable analysis (Table 4.1). Ordinal and nominal variables cannot be used with any of these techniques without transforming the variables.

4.2 What should I do with my ordinal and nominal independent variables?

Don't despair. Ordinal and nominal independent variables can easily be incorporated into all three multivariable models by transforming them into multiple dichotomous variables. This process is usually called "dummying" by epidemiologists and biostatisticians. However, the term "dummying" and "dummy variables" are slang. In manuscripts, refer to this process as creating multiple categorical variables (if you refer to it as dummying, you may, as I did, receive complaints from the reviewers of your article).

Ethnicity is probably the most common nominal variable in clinical research. Obviously, there is no numeric ordering of different ethnicities, let alone a fixed interval between them. Therefore, ethnicity is either dichotomized (e.g., white/nonwhite) or (better) is represented as several dichotomous variables in multivariable analysis. Below I have represented ethnicity as five dichotomous variables:

African-American (yes/no),
Latino/Hispanic (yes/no),
Asian/Pacific Islander (yes/no),

TABLE 4.1

Independent variables and multivariable analysis.

Type of independent variable	Example of independent variable	Multiple linear regression	Multiple logistic regression	Proportional hazards analysis
Interval	Age, blood pressure	Yes	Yes	Yes
Dichotomous	Gender	Yes	Yes	Yes
Ordinal	Cancer stage	No	No	No
Nominal	Ethnicity	No	No	No

Native American (yes/no),
Other nonwhite (yes/no).

What happened to persons who are white/Caucasian? When you represent a nominal variable as several dichotomous variables in multivariable analysis you need one variable less than the number of categories of your variable. Why? To answer this question, think about it from the computer's point of view. If you create five dichotomous variables, all of which are either 1 (yes) or 0 (no), the computer will see six patterns as shown in Table 4.2.

We don't create a variable white/Caucasian because it is represented by the other five variables (zero on all five variables). In multivariable analysis, this is called a reference or referent variable.

I deliberately chose ethnicity as an example of a nominal variable because how you choose to code it will depend on your study population. For example, in a small clinical study performed in the southeast of the United States, there may be very few Native Americans or Asian/Pacific Islanders. If a group represents less than 5% of the total sample, creating a variable for that group may not carry much statistically important information. In this case you might only create variables for the larger ethnic groups and then have a group that is "other." For example, your variables would be African-American (yes/no), Latino/Hispanic (yes/no), and other nonwhite ethnicity (yes/no), with white as the reference group.

Although decreasing the number of groups may prevent having dichotomous variables that convey little information, grouping people of different ethnicities in one group may not adequately represent the

TABLE 4.2
Creation of multiple dichotomous variables to represent a nominal independent variable

	African-American	Latino/Hispanic	Asian/Pacific Islander	Native American	Other nonwhite
African-American	1	0	0	0	0
Latino/Hispanic	0	1	0	0	0
Asian/Pacific Islander	0	0	1	0	0
Native American	0	0	0	1	0
Other nonwhite	0	0	0	0	1
White/Caucasian	0	0	0	0	0

data. Even if you retain the category "Asian/Pacific Islander" remember that this category contains more than a dozen disparate cultures, each with their own language, traditions, and genetic composition, all of which could affect the development of disease. As with all really hard questions in multivariable analyses, the question of how to code ethnicity is not a statistical question. The best way to group a nominal independent variable such as ethnicity will depend on the research question, the distribution of the nominal variable (how many people are in each group), and the relationship between the different categories of the nominal variable and the outcome.

The process of creating multiple dichotomous variables has other uses besides allowing you to incorporate ordinal and nominal variables. It also works in the case of interval variables, for which the relationship between the untransformed interval-independent variable and the outcome does not fit the assumptions of the model. This issue is dealt with in greater detail in Section 5.5.

As discussed in Section 3.2, some variables, while technically ordinal, operate as if they were interval. Just as you can use certain ordinal variables as dependent variables in multiple linear regression, you can use such variables as independent variables in all three types of analysis, as long as they fulfill the assumptions of your model.

> ✓ **TIP**
>
> The best way to group a nominal variable will depend on the research question, the distribution of the nominal variable, and the bivariate relationship between the nominal variable and the outcome.

5

Assumptions of Multiple Linear Regression, Multiple Logistic Regression, and Proportional Hazards Analysis

5.1 What are the assumptions of multiple linear regression, multiple logistic regression, and proportional hazards analysis?

As shown in Table 5.1, the assumptions underlying the three multivariable models differ somewhat with respect to what is being modeled, the relationship of multiple independent variables to outcome, the relationship of an interval-independent variable to the outcome, the distribution of the outcome variable, and the variance of the outcome variable. These assumptions are explained in this chapter.

Proportional hazards analysis has two additional assumptions with regard to censored observations and relative hazards over time (referred to as the proportionality assumption). These are dealt with in Sections 7.4 and 10.10, respectively.

5.2 What is being modeled in multiple linear regression, multiple logistic regression, and proportional hazards analysis?

In multiple linear regression, as the independent variable increases (or decreases) the mean or expected value of the outcome increases (or decreases) in a linear fashion. Many clinical situations fit this linear assumption.

For example, Figure 5.1 shows the relationship between B_{12} levels and pneumococcal antibody levels following receipt of pneumococcal vaccination among elderly persons.[29] Each square represents an

---

[29] Fata, F.T., Herzlich, B.C., Schiffman, G., et al. "Impaired antibody responses to pneumococcal polysaccharide in elderly patients with low serum vitamin B_{12} levels." *Ann. Intern. Med.* 1996; 124:299–304.

TABLE 5.1
Multivariable model assumptions.

	Multiple linear regression	Multiple logistic regression	Proportional hazards analysis
What is being modeled?	The mean value of the outcome.	The logarithm of the odds of the outcome (referred to as *logit*).	The logarithm of the relative hazard.
Relationship of multiple indepen-dent variables to outcome	The mean value of outcome changes *linearly* with multiple indepen-dent variables.	The logit of the outcome changes *linearly* with multiple indepen-dent variables.	The logarithm of the relative hazard changes *linearly* with multiple indepen-dent variables.
Relationship of an interval-indepen-dent variable to outcome	The mean value of outcome changes *linearly* with each unit change in interval-indepen-dent variable.	The logit of outcome changes *linearly* with each unit change in interval-indepen-dent variable.	The logarithm of the relative hazard changes *linearly* with each unit change in interval-indepen-dent variable.
Distribution of outcome variable	Normal	Binomial	None specified
Variance of outcome variable	Equal ground the mean	Depends only on the mean	None specified
Censored observations	Not applicable	Not applicable	Censored cases have the same time to outcome as noncensored cases (Section 7.4).
Relative hazard over time	Not applicable	Not applicable	Constant (Section 10.10)

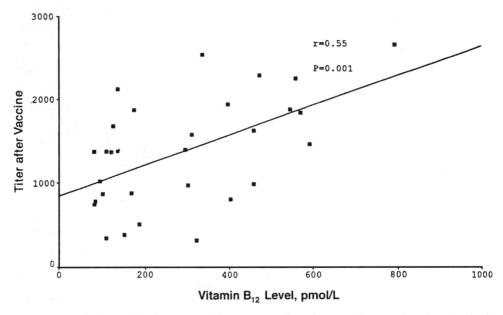

Figure 5.1. Linear association between vitamin B$_{12}$ levels and pneumococcal antibody titers after pneumococcal vaccination. Reproduced with permission from: Fata, F.T., et al. "Impaired antibody responses to pneumococcal polysaccharide in elderly patients with low serum vitamin B$_{12}$ levels." *Ann. Intern. Med.* 1996; 124:299–304.

observation (a person) and their vitamin B$_{12}$ level (the independent variable) and their antibody titer after vaccine (the dependent variable). Although arbitrary, the convention is to show the independent variable on the *x* axis and the dependent variable on the *y* axis.

The linear regression line shows the best single representation of the data. But note that only two points actually fall on the line and many points are not even that close to the line. Statistical models are, at best, approximations of data. The linear assumption does not mean that all observations fit a linear model; it means that a line is a good representation of the fact that as vitamin B$_{12}$ levels increase, the levels of antibodies also increase.

In clinical research the outcome is often a disease or disease state that cannot be measured on an interval scale: cancer, stroke, heart attack, death. In Section 3.1, I indicated that logistic regression, rather than linear regression, is used for dichotomous outcomes. Although this is true, you can use linear regression for dichotomous outcomes. It just doesn't work as well in most cases. Understanding why will lead us to the advantages of the logistic regression model.

ASSUMPTIONS

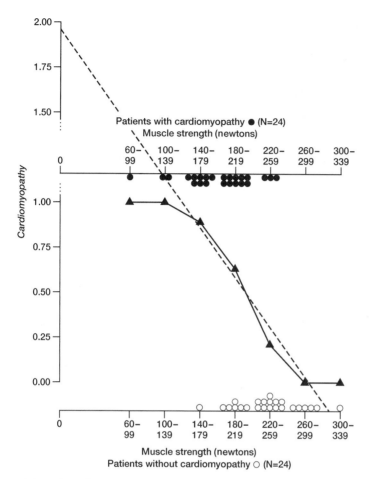

Figure 5.2. Z-shaped association between skeletal muscle strength and presence of cardiomyopathy among alcoholics. The closed circles are patients with cardiomyopathy and the open circles are patients without cardiomyopathy. The triangles show the observed proportion of patients with cardiomyopathy at different levels of muscle strength. Data are from Fernandez-Sola, J., Estruch, R., Grau, J.M., Pare J.C., Rubin, E., Urbano-Marquez, A. "The relationship of alcoholic myopathy to cardiomyopathy." *Ann. Intern. Med.* 1994; 120:529–36.

In Figure 5.2, we see the association between skeletal muscle strength (measured in the deltoid muscle) and presence of cardio-myopathy among alcoholics.[30] You can see that at low levels of muscle

[30] Fernandez-Sola, J., Estruch, R., Grau, J.M., Pare, J.C., Rubin, E, Urbano-Marquez, A. "The relationship of alcoholic myopathy to cardiomyopathy." *Ann. Intern. Med.* 1994; 120:529–36.

strength (left-hand side of the curve), there are several closed circles (representing patients with cardiomyopathy) while there are no open circles (patients with normal cardiac function). In contrast, at high levels of muscle strength (right-hand side of the curve) there are many open circles and few closed circles, reflecting that patients without cardiomyopathy have normal muscle strength. The triangles indicate the probability of cardiomyopathy at different levels of muscle strength. The curve connecting the triangles shows that at intermediate levels of muscle strength, there is a rapidly decreasing proportion of patients with cardiomyopathy as muscle strength increases.

The probability of cardiomyopathy, as with any event, cannot be less than zero or greater than one. The value of the logistic function is that it incorporates this assumption. Logistic regression models the logit of the outcome. The logit is the natural logarithm of the odds of the outcome. The odds of the outcome is the probability of having the outcome divided by the probability of not having the outcome. Whereas the logit can take on any value from minus to plus infinity, the probability, which is the inverse of the logit, can only take on values of zero to one. This gives the logistic function an S or Z shape (depending on which way the outcome variable is configured). As you can see in Figure 5.2, this shape fits the data. Note that as the probability of outcome approaches zero or one, further increases or decreases in the independent variable have little effect on the outcome.

I have drawn a linear regression line (the dotted line) so that you can appreciate that a linear function could be used to model the data. But there are problems. Cardiomyopathy is either present or not. Yet the line would predict that a patient with muscle strength of less than 100 newtons would have a value greater than one on the cardiomyopathy variable. The line would also indicate that a patient with muscle strength of 300 newtons or greater would have a negative value on the cardiomyopathy variable. Obviously, these values are impossible.

Although this S- or Z-shaped function is useful, remember that it is still just a model. The curve I have drawn in Figure 5.2 is based on the actual data. The estimated curve would be of a similar shape but would not go exactly through the boxes. We will take up the issue of how to assess how well the shape of the model fits the observed data in Section 9.2.

Based on Table 3.1 it would be logical to assume that proportional hazards analysis models time to event. While logical, this is incorrect. Proportional hazards analysis models the natural logarithm of the relative hazard. The relative hazard is the ratio of time to outcome given a particular risk factor to time to outcome when the risk factor is not present. For example, persons who smoke may have six times the risk of heart attack as persons who do not smoke. The fact that the underlying time to outcome (in this example, heart attack) is not modeled is one of the features that gives proportional hazards analysis its tremendous flexibility.

5.3 What is the relationship of multiple independent variables to outcome in multiple linear regression, multiple logistic regression, and proportional hazards analysis?

In Section 5.2, we reviewed what was being modeled by each of the three models. However, in the examples, for the sake of simplicity, I illustrated the principles with a single independent variable. Of course, the whole point of multivariable analysis is to include multiple independent variables. What is the relationship of multiple independent variables to outcome? As you can see from Table 5.1 all three models assume a linear component to the relationship of multiple independent variables to outcome, but the relationship is linear on different scales.

With multiple linear regression, the expected value of the outcome changes linearly with the weighted sum of the independent variables. With multiple logistic regression, the logit changes linearly with the weighted sum of the independent variables. With proportional hazards analysis, the logarithm of the relative hazard changes linearly with the weighted sum of the independent variables. In all three models, the weights are determined by the strength of the independent variables in accounting for the outcome.

5.4 What is the relationship of an interval-independent variable to the outcome in multiple linear regression, multiple logistic regression, and proportional hazards analysis?

As you will remember, each unit of an interval variable is equal and quantifiable. All three multivariable methods assume that a unit change anywhere on the scale of an interval variable will have a linear effect on outcome. However, just as with multiple independent variables, the relationship is linear on different scales.

In the case of multiple linear regression, the change in the mean value of the outcome is modeled as the sum of the unit changes of the interval-independent variable. With logistic regression, the logit of the outcome is modeled as the sum of the unit changes of the interval-independent variable. With proportional hazards analysis, the logarithm of the relative hazard is modeled as the sum of the unit changes of the interval-independent variable.

The linearity assumption for linear regression is best tested by constructing a scatter plot of your raw independent variable versus your outcome variable. Look back at Figure 5.1. It is a typical scatter plot showing a linear relationship between two interval variables, with higher values of B_{12} being associated with higher titers after vaccine.

Sometimes a scatter plot will not show a linear relationship. Instead, you may see one of the shapes in Figure 5.3: logarithmic, antilogarithmic, curvilinear (**U**-shape, upside down **U**–shape, **J**-shape), and threshold. If you see a nonlinear relationship, you cannot proceed with linear regression without transforming the variable (Section 5.5).

In the case of multiple logistic regression and proportional hazards analysis, you cannot assess the linear assumption by making a simple scatter plot. This is because the linear relationship does not exist on a simple arithmetic scale. Instead, to assess whether an interval variable fits the linear assumption of logistic regression or proportional hazards analysis, categorize the variable into multiple dichotomous variables (Section 4.2) of equal units on the variable's scale. So, for example, if the variable you are testing is age, and the age of your subjects ranges from 20 to 79, have age 20–29 be your reference group. Then create variables 30–39 (yes/no), 40–49 (yes/no), 50–59 (yes/no), 60–69 (yes/no), and 70–79 (yes/no). If you would have too few subjects being yes in these decade categories, you can group them into 20-year periods.

Perform the logistic or proportional hazards analysis with these several dichotomous variables. Each variable will have an estimated coefficient. The coefficient for the reference group is, by definition, 0. Graph the coefficient against the midpoint of each dichotomous variable (e.g., 35 years for the variable that represents the 30–39 group). The graph will show you the relationship between your independent and outcome variable. If you have a linear effect, the coefficients will steadily increase (or decrease) as you go from one age group to another, and you will get a straight line (as shown in Figure 5.4). Alternatively, your graph may appear like one of the nonlinear relationships in Figure 5.3.

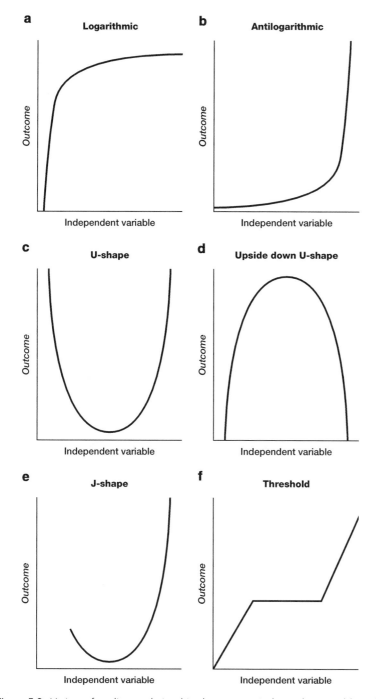

Figure 5.3. Variety of nonlinear relationships between an independent variable and an outcome.

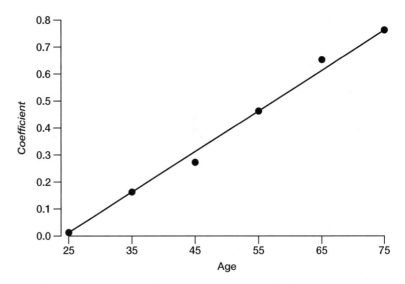

Figure 5.4. Coefficients graphed against age form a straight line.

Even without graphing, if you have a linear effect, the numeric difference between the coefficients of each successive group should be about equal (e.g., the numeric difference between the coefficient of the 30–39 group and the coefficient of the 20–29 group will be equal to the difference between the coefficient of the 40–49 variable and the 30–39 variable). Remember, of course, they are not going to be exactly equal (just as the points do not fall exactly on a straight line). The important issue is whether the data can be reasonably expressed as a linear relationship.

This technique can be used to determine whether a linear relationship exists between an independent variable and an outcome variable after adjustment for potential confounders (Section 10.3). Besides being useful for testing a linear association, this technique is also useful for demonstrating a linear dose response curve between an independent variable and outcome.[31]

With logistic regression analysis, there is another method of assessing the linearity assumption of an interval-independent variable. It requires grouping your interval-independent variable data into

---

[31] If you are unfamiliar with multiple logistic regression and proportional hazards analysis, this section will make more sense to you after you have read Section 9.3 on interpretation of coefficients. For a more detailed explanation of this technique see Hosmer, D.W., Lemeshow, S. *Applied Logistic Regression*. New York: Wiley, 1989, pp. 95–7.

categories that preserve the interval nature of the variable (e.g., 1 = ages 20–29, 2 = ages 30–39, 3 = ages 40–49, etc.) and are large enough to provide a reasonable number of outcomes in each category. You can then perform a simple cross-tabulation of your independent variable and outcome. The cross-tabulation table should show a steadily increasing (or decreasing) proportion of outcomes as you increase (or decrease) along the levels of your interval-independent variable. The chi-square for trend test should be significant.

5.5 What if my interval-independent variable does not have a linear relationship with my outcome?

In clinical research, interval-independent variables often have the kind of nonlinear relationships with outcome that are shown in Figure 5.3. If you treat these nonlinear relationships as if they were linear, your results may appear sensible. No alarms will go off, your computer will not melt down, and your printout will not look like number salad. Your results may show no relationship between the independent variable and the outcome or may show a weak linear relationship, especially if there are a large number of points along the scale where the relationship is linear.

Modeling such variables as if they were linear clearly is not right. However, don't be discouraged if your variable does not fit the linear relationship assumed by your model. This observation provides valuable information and by transforming the variable you will still be able to keep it in your model.

If changes in value at the high end of your independent variable have less impact on your outcome variable than changes at the lower end (as indicated by a steadily decreasing slope with the high end of the independent variable asymptotically approaching a horizontal level as in Figure 5.3a), a logarithmic transformation of the independent variable (the logarithm of the variable) may linearize the trend. The natural logarithm is used more often than logarithm to the base 10, although both may linearize the effect. Remember that with either logarithmic transformation, values for the variable must be positive (i.e., you cannot take the logarithm of zero or negative numbers). If your scale has a true zero you can still use a logarithmic transformation by adding one to all values.

If changes in value at the high end of your independent variable have a greater impact on your outcome variable than changes at the lower end (as indicated by a steadily increasing slope as in Figure 5.3b),

> **✓ TIP**
>
> If changes in value at the high end of your independent variable have less impact on your outcome variable than changes at the lower end, try a logarithmic transformation of the independent variable to linearize the trend.

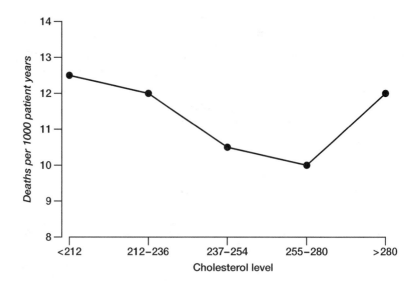

Figure 5.5. Relationship between cholesterol level and all cause mortality among 1,102 women. Adapted with permission from: Isles, C.G., et al. "Plasma cholesterol, coronary heart disease, and cancer in the Renfrew and Paisley survey." *Br. Med. J.* 1989;298:920–4. Copyright BMJ Publishing Group.

> **✓ TIP**
>
> If changes in value at the high end of your independent variable have a greater impact on your outcome variable than changes at the lower end, try an antilogarithm transformation of the independent variable to linearize the trend.

an antilogarithm transformation (i.e., e^x or 10^x) of the independent variable may linearize the trend. Logarithmic or antilogarithmic transformations can be made of the independent or dependent variable.[32]

In Figure 5.5, we see the **U**-shaped relationship between cholesterol level and all-cause mortality in a sample of 1,102 women.[33] Mortality is highest for women with the lowest and the highest values of cholesterol. When the investigators treated cholesterol as an interval variable, there was no significant relationship between cholesterol level and mortality, because the two trends statistically cancel each out. Treating cholesterol as an interval variable misses the vital information contained in the curvilinear relationship: High cholesterol levels are associated with increased mortality from coronary artery disease, whereas low levels of cholesterol are associated with increased mortality from cancer and other causes.

---

[32] Other mathematical transformations are possible: See Armitage, P., Berry, G., *Statistical Methods in Medical Research* (2nd ed.). Oxford: Blackwell Scientific Publications, 1987, pp. 358–68.

[33] Isles, C.G., Hole, D.J., Gillis, C.R., Hawthorne, V.M., Lever, A.F. "Plasma cholesterol, coronary heart disease, and cancer in the Renfrew and Paisley survey." *Br. Med. J.* 1989; 298:920–4.

ASSUMPTIONS

As you can tell from Figure 5.3, a **J**-shaped curve is just like a **U**-shaped curve with a few missing data points. What can you do when your bivariate plots show a **U**- or **J**-shaped relationship? You have two possible solutions. You can include a quadratic form of the variable in addition to the untransformed value of the variable. To create the quadratic form of the variable first subtract out the mean of the variable: (value of X – mean of X for sample)^2. The untransformed variable must be in the equation because the quadratic term is comparing extremes to the mean of the untransformed variable. Large differences from the mean in either direction cause the term to be statistically significant. If the relationship is **U**- or **J**-shaped both terms will be statistically significant in your model. A limitation of this technique is that it is hard to describe to your reader how a unit change in the independent variable affects the outcome (because a unit change affects the outcome through two variables – each with a different relationship with the outcome.)

A more common solution to modeling a curvilinear relationship is to create multiple dichotomous variables as you would to incorporate a nominal variable into your analysis (Section 4.2). This allows each category to be its own independent variable and have its own relationship to the outcome. One limitation of this strategy is that the choice of cutoffs can be somewhat arbitrary. If you choose the cutoff points to maximize the association between an independent variable and the outcome, you will overestimate the association between these variables in the population. Therefore, in choosing cutoffs you should either use natural cutoffs (e.g., decades of age, systolic blood pressure <140 mm, 140–159 mm, 160–179 mm, etc.) or divide the sample into equal sample sizes by the independent variable (terciles, quartiles, quintiles of values of the independent variable).

A disadvantage of choosing natural cutoffs, such as decades of age, is that the cutoffs may divide the sample into groups with unequal sample sizes. For example, if you divide your sample into decades of age, you may only have 2% of your sample as "yes" on the variable 80–89 years. If the number of persons who are yes on this variable is too small, the variable will not be meaningful in the analysis. In comparison, if you choose cutoffs that provide equal sample sizes then the distributions of the multiple dichotomous variables will be equal. For example, let's assume you divide the sample into terciles of age and make the youngest people the reference group. One dichotomous variable will have a "yes" value for a third of the sample (the middle-aged people) and a "no" value for two thirds of the sample (the youngest

> ✓ **TIP**
>
> Model a curvilinear relationship by creating multiple dichotomous variables.

and oldest persons); the other dichotomous variable will also have a "yes" value for a third of the sample (the oldest persons) and a "no" value for two thirds of the sample (the youngest and the middle-aged persons).

The disadvantage of using cutoffs based on equal sample sizes is that the results may not sound as compelling because you lose the units of the independent variable. Which of the following sounds more compelling? Persons in the highest tercile of age are three times more likely to die than persons in the lowest tercile of age or persons aged 70–89 years are three times more likely to die than persons aged 30–49 years. The latter sounds more compelling. Don't you think?

Besides curvilinear relationships, threshold effects are commonly seen in clinical research. As you can see by looking at Figure 5.3f, threshold effects, which often look like a step function, cannot be modeled as linear. Instead it is best to create multiple dichotomous variables. The curve in Figure 5.3f has essentially three segments (two steep sections and one flat section). You could model this as two dichotomous variables with one of the segments serving as the reference category.

Creation of multiple dichotomous variables allows incorporation of any nonlinear effect. Because they allow each category its own association with outcome, multiple dichotomous variables will work even when other transformations do not. For example, Phibbs and colleagues wanted to use a linear function to describe the association between birth weight and mortality.[34] However, the association between birth weight and mortality did not fit a linear model, even when they performed logarithmic, reciprocal, and quadratic transformations. They therefore created multiple dichotomous variables.

One downside of multiple dichotomous variables is that they increase the number of variables in your model. This can be a problem if you do not have a large enough sample size (Section 7.1).

Armed with the knowledge of how to transform variables, what would you do with the data from a study of the incidence of severe cerebral outcome (deficit in intellectual function, memory deficit, or seizure) following coronary bypass surgery shown in Figure 5.6?[35] You will note that the incidence of severe adverse cerebral outcome does

> ✓ **TIP**
>
> Creation of multiple dichotomous variables allows incorporation of any nonlinear effect.

[34] Phibbs, C.S., Bronstein, J.M., Buxton, E., Phibbs, R.H. "The effects of patient volume and level of care at the hospital of birth on neonatal mortality." *JAMA* 1996; 276:1054–9.

[35] Roach, G.W., Kanchuger, M., Mangano, C.M., et al. "Adverse cerebral outcomes after coronary bypass surgery." *N. Engl. J. Med.* 1996; 335:1857–63.

ASSUMPTIONS

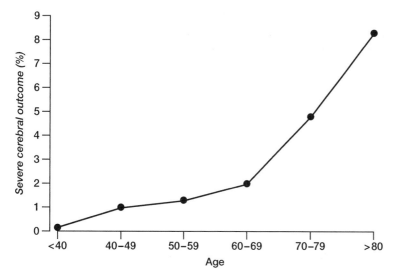

Figure 5.6. Relationship between age and incidence of severe cerebral outcome. Adapted with permission from Roach, G.W., et al. "Adverse cerebral outcomes after coronary bypass surgery." *N. Engl. J. Med.* 1996; 335:1857–63. Copyright © 1996 Massachusetts Medical Society. All rights reserved.

not increase linearly with age. The incidence increases noticeably from those <40 years (0%) to those 40–49 years (1%). Then the risk increases slightly among those 50–59 (1.3%) and 60–69 years (2%). Finally, the risk increases more than twofold for those 70–79 (4.8%) and almost another twofold for those ≥80 (8.3%) years of age. Because of the flat part of the curve, the only transformation that would really fit the data would be multiple dichotomous variables. If you made the <40 year group the reference group, the variables representing age 70–79 (yes/no) and >80 years (yes/no) would have large coefficients that were different from one another, whereas the coefficients for the variables 40–49 (yes/no), 50–59 (yes/no), and 60–69 (yes/no) would be small and similar to one another.

Although Figure 5.6 showing the nonlinear relationship between age and incidence of severe cerebral outcome was printed in the article, the authors did not transform the variable. In their proportional hazards analysis, the authors used age as an interval variable in decades. The relative hazard associated with each additional decade was 1.75. Looking back at Figure 5.6 you can see why. An increase of 1.75 underestimates the effect of a ten-year increase in age in the range of 60 to over 80 years of age, but it overestimates the impact of a ten-year difference in the less than 40 to 60 year range.

This example illustrates an important point: Your multivariable analysis can look and be sensible, even if the variable does not fit the linear gradient. Are you surprised that I say the result is sensible? What I mean is, if you had to give a single estimate of the effect of age on incidence of severe cerebral outcome, 1.75 per decade would be the best estimate. It just happens that this estimate is not a very good representation of the true impact of age on the risk of outcome over the life span.

It is easier to determine whether an independent variable is linearly related to an outcome variable in a bivariate analysis than in a multivariable analysis. For this reason, you should evaluate the linear nature of the variable in bivariate analysis. If the variable is linear in bivariate analysis you may treat it that way in multivariable analysis. However, ideally you should perform additional tests to see how well the variable fulfills the linear assumption in the multivariable model (Sections 10.2 and 10.3).

5.6 Assuming that my interval-independent variable fits a linear assumption is there any reason to group it into interval categories or create multiple dichotomous variables?

Even when an interval-independent variable, such as age, blood pressure, or cholesterol, fits the linear assumption it is often not left in its original interval form. There are several reasons for this.

For one thing, if you have a small sample size (e.g., 100 persons) it may be difficult to evaluate whether an interval variable (e.g., age) fits the linear assumption unless you group it into categories. Left ungrouped your model will assume that the difference in the likelihood of outcome between a subject age 55 and a subject age 57 is the same as that between a subject age 61 and a subject age 63. Yet you may have no one or just one or two persons in your entire sample with these ages. Also, your audience is likely to be more interested in the impact of ten years on outcome, than the impact of a single year (which is likely to be very small for most diseases).

✓ T I P

When grouping interval variables maintain the interval nature of the scale.

When grouping an interval variable maintain the interval nature of the scale (e.g., group age by decades). This will allow you to retain the advantages of an interval scale (because the difference between being 20–29, 30–39, and 40–49, etc. is the same – 10 years). Yet, you will be better able to assess whether the variable fits the assumptions of the statistical model and you will be able to report a more meaningful result.

ASSUMPTIONS

Sometimes researchers create multiple dichotomous variables even though the variable approximates a linear relationship. The reason is that creation of multiple dichotomous variables is a more conservative strategy. Since a linear relationship is not assumed, you do not have to prove to your readers (or your reviewers!) that the linear assumption is fulfilled. If you have a sufficient sample size to afford creation of several dichotomous variables, this strategy may work well for you. On the negative side, a weak linear trend may be statistically significant if left as an interval variable, but when represented as multiple dichotomous variables, it no longer appears to be statistically significant because none of the variables themselves are significant.

5.7 What are the assumptions about the distribution of the outcome and the variance?

Multiple linear regression assumes a normal distribution and equal variance around the mean.[36] A normal distribution has a bell shape. To fulfill this condition your outcome variable should have a bell-shaped curve for any value of your independent variable. This is shown in Figure 5.7a. Note that for each of the three values of the independent variable (X_1, X_2, and X_3), the range of values of the dependent variable forms a bell-shaped curve. Equal variance means that the spread of dependent variable values (indicated by arrows) from the mean (indicated with a dotted line) is equal for each value of X. This is the case in Figure 5.7a.

> Multiple linear regression assumes a normal distribution and equal variance around the mean.

If you have an interval-independent variable, it is easier to assess these assumptions if you group the independent variable into a few groups. So, for example, in Figure 5.7a, X_1, X_2, and X_3 may represent a range of values (e.g., age 20–39 years, 40–59 years, 60–69 years.)

Figure 5.7b shows a bivariate relationship that does not fulfill the assumptions of normal distribution or equal variance. Note that the values of the dependent variable for X_1 and X_2 both produce normal shaped curves, but the variance is not equal. It is much smaller for values of X_1 than for values of X_2. At X_3 we see a curve with a skewed distribution (long tail). This curve does not have a bell-shaped

---

[36] The technical term for equal variance for any value of X is homoscedasticity. "Homo" meaning same and "scedastic" from the Greek word "to scatter." For a more detailed explanation of these and the other assumptions of linear regression, see Kleinbaum, D.G., Kupper, L.L., Muller, K.E. *Applied Regression Analysis and Other Multivariable Methods* (2nd ed.). Boston: PWS-Kent, 1988, pp. 44–9.

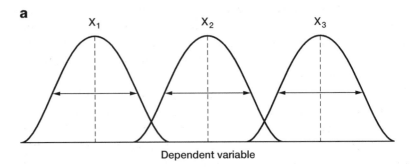

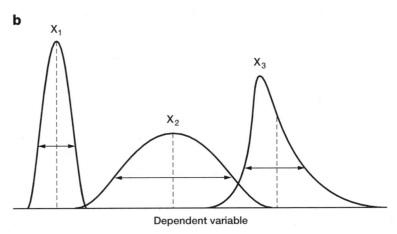

Dependent variable

Figure 5.7. Plots of an interval dependent variable at three different values of the independent variable X. In Figure 5.7a, the assumptions of normal distribution and equal variance are fulfilled because at all three values of X, the curves are bell-shaped and the spread from the mean (indicated by arrows) is equal. In Figure 5.7b these assumptions are not met. The assumption of normal distribution is violated because the distribution of values for X_3 does not form a bell-shaped curved. The equal variance assumption is invalid because the spread of values from the mean is different for the three values of X.

distribution and the variance is not equal to the other two curves. Therefore, the relationship between this independent and dependent variable does not fit the assumptions of normal distribution or equal variance. Conceptually you should think of the assumptions of normal distribution and equal variance as two separate conditions, although, in practice (as with this example) variables departing from one assumption often depart from the other.

Some investigators mistakenly believe that they can evaluate the assumption of normal distribution by assessing only the univariate characteristics of the variable. In other words, they print a histogram for all values of X. If the distribution is bell shaped they conclude that

ASSUMPTIONS

it fulfills the assumption of normal distribution. However, as explained above, the assumption of normal distribution and equal variance apply to each level of the independent variable, not all values together. Nonetheless, a simple histogram of all your independent variables is a useful first step.

If you find that the univariate distribution of your variable has a significant departure from the bell-shaped curve, it is likely that it will violate the assumption of normal distribution and equal variance in bivariate analysis. Since it is easier to review a univariate distribution than a bivariate association, this procedure alerts you to which variables to watch especially carefully in your analysis. In addition to eyeballing the histogram, you can use one of many statistical packages to provide you with a normal probability plot, which should approximate a line if the data are normally distributed. The statistics skewness and kurtosis when high also indicate that the data do not fit a normal distribution, but these are less informative than looking at the histogram.

Besides alerting you to potential violations of the assumptions of normal distribution and equal variance, printing histograms of your dependent and independent variables is a necessary step in cleaning your data. Histograms allow you to detect implausible values (e.g., age of 120 years) and help identify gaps in your values. If, for example, you have few observations of persons older than 60 years of age, your results will not necessarily generalize to this older group. Univariate statistics will also help you to detect extreme (but plausible) values (outliers) that might affect your results, such as two octogenarians. If you happen to have two octogenarians and they happen to have extreme values on your outcome variable, they may unduly influence your results (Section 10.4).

Now that you have read all of the above theory and considered what a pain it would be to perform the recommended analysis for each of your independent variables, I am happy to tell you, that if your sample size is large (greater than 100), you can assume that the assumption of normal distribution is met (assuming you do not have any unduly influential points). We have the central limit theorem to thank for this great gift, the details of which are beyond the scope of this book.

Only significant departures from equal variance are likely to affect your results. The usual effect would be to decrease the power of your analysis to demonstrate an association between your independent and dependent variables.

> ✓ **T I P**
>
> Run histograms for all your variables. They will alert you to: a) Potential violations of normality and equal variance, b) implausible values, c) gaps in your values, and d) extreme values.

> ✓ **T I P**
>
> If your sample size is large (greater than 100), you can assume that the assumption of normality is met.

With logistic regression, the dependent variable is assumed to have a binomial distribution. A binomial distribution describes the number of successes or failures (e.g., yes or no; survival or death) in a series of *independent* trials. Independent trials mean that the outcome for one subject is independent of the outcome for another subject. In other words, the outcomes are not clustered due to being from the same individuals, families, or medical practices. There are methods for dealing with clustered effects (Sections 12.2 and 12.3). The variances in logistic regression are assumed to depend only on the mean.

With proportional hazards analysis the distribution of the outcome and the variance is unspecified (i.e., no assumption is made).

5.8 What should I do if I find significant violations of the assumptions of normal distribution and equal variance in my multiple linear regression analysis?

> **✓ TIP**
>
> If you find significant departures from the assumptions of normality and equal variance try transforming the independent or dependent variable.

If you find *significant* departures from the assumptions of normal distribution and equal variance what should you do? You can attempt to transform either the independent or dependent variable so that the relationship fits these assumptions. Commonly performed transformations are the natural logarithm, the square root, the reciprocal, the square, and the arcsin.[37]

Once you have transformed the variable you need to repeat the bivariate relationship to see if indeed the variable more closely fits the assumptions of your model.

Our ultimate concern will be whether these assumptions are met on a multivariable level, in other words, when all independent variables are in the model. Unfortunately, it is harder to illustrate these principles with multiple independent variables. Nonetheless, there are tests that can be performed to assess these assumptions on the multivariable level. They are dealt with in Section 10.2.

[37] For a fuller discussion of these transformations see Kleinbaum, D.G., Kupper, L.L., and Muller, K.E. *Applied Regression Analysis and Other Multivariable Methods* (2nd ed.). Boston: PWS-Kent, 1988, pp. 220–1.

6

Relationship of Independent Variables to One Another

6.1 Does it matter if my independent variables are related to each other?

As discussed in Section 1.1, the strength of multivariable analysis is its ability to determine how multiple independent variables, which are related to one another, are related to an outcome. We would not need multivariable analysis to determine the independent effect of exercise on mortality if it weren't for the fact that exercise, smoking, age, hypertension, and cholesterol level were all related to each other and the outcome of interest. Multivariable analysis helps us to separate the effects of these different variables on outcomes such as mortality.

However, if two variables are so closely correlated that if you know the value for one variable you know the value of the other, multivariable analysis cannot separately assess the impact of these two variables on the outcome. This problem is called multicollinearity. I can best illustrate it with an extreme example.

> ⏵ **DEFINITION**
>
> *Multicollinearity* occurs when two or more variables are so closely related to one another that the model may not be able to reliably assess the independent contribution of each variable.

Let's say you were studying factors that affected length of hospital stay among patients with pneumonia. At your hospital, to accommodate the different preferences of the staff, the nurses record patient's temperature in both Fahrenheit and Celsius. When you do your medical abstraction, you record both Fahrenheit and Celsius temperatures. If you entered both variables in a model assessing length of stay, your model would be incorrect, and you would get an error message or unpredictable answers. This is because temperature in Celsius and temperature in Fahrenheit is the same variable even though the numbers are different. There is a simple mathematical conversion from one to the other: Celsius = (Fahrenheit − 32) 0.56.

Your model cannot possibly assess the independent contribution of temperature in Fahrenheit and in Celsius because they are really the same variable. However, unless you make a mistake and include two variables that really are the same variable (such as temperature in Fahrenheit and in Celsius) it would be very unlikely to have a situation where two variables are exactly correlated with one another. A more likely scenario is to have variables that are not sufficiently different for the model to distinguish them. For example, Phibbs and colleagues found that birth weight and gestational age were too closely related to include both in their analysis of neonatal mortality.[38]

6.2   How do I assess whether my variables are multicollinear?

The correlation coefficient (also called Pearson correlation or *r*) is a bivariate statistic that measures how strongly two variables are related to one another. The correlation coefficient assumes the relationship between the two variables is linear. It can range from −1 to 1. When the coefficient is −1 or 1 the two variables change together exactly (i.e., knowing one variable tells you the value of the other variable). The only difference between −1 and 1 is that the negative sign indicates that the two variables change exactly together in opposite directions (i.e., as one goes higher the other goes lower). Zero indicates that there is no relationship whatsoever. If you square the correlation coefficient and multiply by 100 you get a measure of how much information the two variables share ranging from 0% to 100%.

The correlation between temperature in Fahrenheit and in Celsius is 1.0. The two variables share 100% of the same information. In contrast, the correlation between vitamin B_{12} level and pneumococcal antibody titer following immunization was found to be 0.55 (Figure 5.1). The two variables share 30% ($.55^2 \times 100 = 30$) of the same information.

To determine how correlated your independent variables are you may run a correlation coefficient matrix with all your proposed independent variables. In general, two variables that are correlated at more than 0.9 will pose problems in your analysis. Variables correlated at less than 0.8 will not pose problems. Variables correlated between 0.8 and 0.9 may cause problems.

---

[38] Phibbs, C.S., Bronstein, J.M., Buston, W., Phibbs, R.H. "The effects of patient volume and level of care at the hospital of birth on neonatal morality." *JAMA* 1996; 276:1054–9.

The problem with a correlation matrix is that it assesses only the relationship between two variables, without adjustment for the other variables. For this reason, most multivariable analysis programs will print out a correlation matrix for the parameter estimates. Since these estimates are adjusted for one another they are a better measure of whether two variables will result in problems of multicollinearity. As with simple correlations, values greater than .9 will cause problems, whereas those between .8 and .9 are in the gray area.

Astute readers will note that these two techniques deal only with the simplest case of multicollinearity, when one independent variable is highly related to a second independent variable. What if a combination of independent variables is highly related to another independent variable? Statistically, this is as problematic as the situation where two variables are highly correlated, but as I am sure you will appreciate, it is harder to diagnose.

In a sense we have already dealt with this concept in Section 4.2 on converting nominal variables into multiple dichotomous variables ("dummy variables"). Look back at Table 4.2. You will recall that I said you did not need to create a variable for white ethnicity because if a subject were 0 (no) on the variables for African-American, Latino, Asian/Pacific Islander, Native American, and other nonwhite ethnicity the subject would be of white ethnicity. What if you didn't read this section and entered into your model a yes/no variable for each ethnicity including white? Then you would have a situation where a combination of independent variables completely accounts for the value of a different independent variable. Prove this to yourself, by correctly answering the following questions:

1. A subject is yes on any one of the five variables: African-American, Latino, Asian Pacific Islander, Native American, or other nonwhite ethnicity. What is the subject's value on the white ethnicity variable?
2. A different subject is no on all five of the variables: African-American, Latino, Asian Pacific Islander, Native American, or other nonwhite ethnicity. What is the subject's value on the white ethnicity variable?

You knew that the answer to the first question was **No** and the answer to the second question was **Yes**, even though I didn't tell you anything about the subject's value on the variable white ethnicity. This is a situation where a combination of variables completely determines the value of another variable. If you entered a variable for white ethnicity, in addition to the others, this would result in spurious results in your multivariable model.

How will you know if a combination of variables accounts for another variable's value? Two related measures of multicollinearity are tolerance and the reciprocal of tolerance, the variance inflation factor. Both tell you how much the regression coefficient for a particular variable is determined by the other independent variables in the model. Small tolerance values, including those below 0.25, are worrisome, and those below 0.10 are serious. As you would expect with a reciprocal value, high values of the variance inflation factor, such as values greater than four, are problematic, whereas values greater than 10 are serious.[39]

Most linear regression programs will print out tolerance or variable inflation factors for each of the independent variables in your model. If the values of some of your variables are worrisome, you will need to do additional analyses to determine which of the other variables in the model is closely related with the problematic variable. This can be done by performing regression analyses using the other variables as independent variables to estimate the value of the problematic variable. This will show you which variables are highly related and enable you to decide which variables to keep in the analysis.

With multiple logistic regression and proportional hazards analysis researchers usually rely on the correlation matrix of the multivariable parameter estimates to determine if there are serious problems with multicollinearity. However, tolerance is a standard for allowing variables to enter into the model; variables with very low tolerance values will not enter (Section 8.12).

6.3   What should I do with multicollinear variables?

If you have variables that are highly related, consider your options:

- omit the variable,
- use an "and/or" clause, or
- create a scale.

If you are going to omit one of the variables, how do you decide which one to delete? Omit the one that has more missing data, has more measurement error, or is less satisfactory in some other way. In the study of neonatal mortality referred to above, the investigators kept birth weight and excluded gestational age. They excluded

[39] For more on measures of multicollinearity and when to worry, see Glantz, S.A., Slinker, B.K. *Primer of Applied Regression and Analysis of Variance.* New York: McGraw-Hill, 1990, pp. 181–99.

✓ **T I P**

If you need to omit a variable, omit the one that has more missing data, has more measurement error, or is less satisfactory in some other way.

RELATIONSHIP OF INDEPENDENT VARIABLES TO ONE ANOTHER

gestational age because compared to birth weight there were more cases with missing data on gestational age and it was less reliably coded. Ironically, as the authors point out, gestational age is theoretically the more important factor in accounting for mortality (because age, not weight, is the deciding factor in reaching certain fetal developmental milestones). Therefore they included two additional variables in their analysis (small for gestational age (yes/no) and large for gestational age (yes/no)) to adjust for the fact that weight might not be an accurate measure of gestational age in some cases.

Using "and/or" clauses works well for correlated variables that represent the same process. For example, if you asked patients with pneumonia whether they had diaphoresis (sweats) or rigors (shaking), these two variables would be expected to be closely correlated since rigors are a more extreme form of diaphoresis. However, some patients who had rigors may not have noticed that they were first diaphoretic; some who were diaphoretic may have taken aspirin thereby preventing the rigor. The new variable could be diaphoresis and/or rigor. Patients who had one or both would be reported as "yes" on this variable; those who had neither would be reported as "no."

Creating scales is a strategy often pursued with psychological and sociologic data. In creating scales, the values of multiple variables for each subject are summated to form a single variable that summarizes the meaning of the separate variables. Researchers may intentionally ask subjects multiple related questions to test the reliability of the subject's responses (i.e., when asked a similar question, using different wording, will subjects answer in the same way?) In this case, the researcher usually plans ahead of time which questions will form a scale. Other times researchers will use factor analysis (Section 7.2. B.2) to determine which questions provide similar information.

These three techniques for dealing with multicollinear variables also work when you need to decrease the number of independent variables in your analysis because of insufficient sample size. However, they will not work for decreasing sample size if your variables are not highly related. A variety of methods for decreasing the number of independent variables are detailed in Section 7.2.

7

Setting Up a Multivariable
Analysis: Subjects

7.1 How many subjects do I need to do multivariable analyses?

The sample size needed for multivariable analysis, as with bivariate analysis, depends on the size of the effect you are trying to demonstrate and the variability of the data. It takes a much larger sample size to show that a risk factor is mildly (but statistically) associated with an outcome (e.g., odds ratio of 1.5) than to show that it is strongly associated with an outcome (e.g., odds ratio of 4.0). The reason is that the smaller the sample size, the larger the confidence intervals. The closer the odds ratio is to 1.0 then the more likely wide confidence intervals are to include one. Similarly, although you can never prove the null hypothesis (i.e., no association: odds ratio of 1.0), the larger the sample size the smaller the chance that you have missed an association that was really present. It also takes a larger sample size to demonstrate a difference between groups on a variable that has a great deal of variability (i.e., a large standard deviation).

Determining the needed sample size is referred to as a power calculation (the power to detect a result). Power calculations for multivariable analysis are complicated and generally require consultation with a biostatistician. Nonetheless, there are a couple of rules of thumb that will hold you in good stead.

First, following the formulas provided in a number of excellent texts,[40] determine the sample size needed for a bivariate analysis. If

[40] For an easy to follow guide see Hulley, S.B., Cummings, S.R. *Designing Clinical Research.* Baltimore: Williams and Wilkins, 1988, pp. 139–50. For a more comprehensive review see Friedman, L.M., Furber, C.E., DeMets, D.L. *Fundamentals of Clinical Trials* (2nd ed.). Littleton, MA: PSG Publishing Co., 1985, pp. 83–107.

your dependent variable is rate of outcome, simplify it to the cumulative proportion of persons experiencing an outcome at a particular point in time (e.g., three years). If your power calculation shows that you do not have enough subjects to demonstrate the effect in bivariate analysis, you definitely will not have enough subjects in your multivariable analysis.

The other useful rule of thumb for multiple logistic regression and proportional hazards analysis is that for every independent variable in your model you need at least ten outcomes.[41] The reason I say ten outcomes for each independent variable, rather than twenty subjects for each independent variable (which would be equivalent if your outcome occurred in half your subjects), is that your model is assessing a particular outcome. In most medical studies, less than half of the subjects experience the outcome (e.g., develop cancer or have a heart attack). If your outcome occurs to only five subjects in your study you may not have enough power to answer your research question even if you have a thousand other subjects in whom the outcome does not occur. This is because the model is determining the likelihood of outcome based on those five people. It does not help you to determine the likelihood of no outcome if this is the larger group. The needed sample size is based on the smaller of the two groups. The reason is that outcome and not outcome are mathematically equivalent: the likelihood of not outcome is simply $1-$ (the likelihood of outcome).

The ten outcomes per variable is just a guideline. Just because your sample size does not meet this criteria does not mean that your study won't appear in the *New England Journal of Medicine* (see Chambers and colleagues, example in Section 7.2.A.3). Conversely, even if you have ten outcomes for each independent variable you still may not have an adequate sample size to answer your study question. For example, you may not have enough subjects in one of the categories of a dichotomous independent variable to study its association with outcome. Just as the sample size depends on the less common outcome state, the sample size to demonstrate that a particular independent variable is

> ✓ **TIP**
>
> If your power calculation shows that you do not have enough subjects for demonstrating the effect in bivariate analysis, you definitely will not have enough subjects to demonstrate the effect in multivariable analysis.

> ✓ **TIP**
>
> For multiple logistic regression and proportional hazards analysis you should have at least ten outcomes for each independent variable in your model.

[41] Peduzzi, P., Concato, J., Kemper, E., Holford, T.R., Feinstein, A.R. "A simulation study of the number of events per variable in logistic regression analysis." *J. Clin. Epidemiol.* 1996; 49:1373–9. Peduzzi, P., Concato, J., Feinstein, A.R., Holford, T.R,. "Importance of events per independent variable in proportional hazards regression analysis II. Accuracy and precision of regression estimates." *J. Clin. Epidemiol.* 1995; 48: 1503–10. Harrell, F.E., Lee, K.L., Matchar, D.B., Reichert, T.A. "Regression models for prognostic prediction: Advantages, problems, and suggested solutions." *Cancer Treat. Rep.* 1985; 69:1071–7.

associated with your outcome will depend on the less common of the values of the dichotomous independent variable.

An example will help to illustrate this principle. Schwarcz and colleagues performed a logistic regression analysis to assess the factors associated with having received pneumocystis prophylaxis prior to a diagnosis of pneumocystis pneumonia (PCP) among HIV-infected persons.[42] The total sample size was 326 persons diagnosed with PCP. Of these, 114 (35%) had received prophylaxis prior to their diagnosis of PCP and 212 (65%) had not. The model included six independent variables. Since the smaller number of outcomes was 114 there would appear to be enough subjects; using our rule of thumb we would need 60 outcomes.

As you can see in Table 7.1, two variables were significantly associated (adjusted P value <0.05) with a lower likelihood of having received prophylaxis in the logistic regression analysis: being nonwhite and being uninsured. Note that the confidence intervals for these two variables exclude one and are reasonably narrow.

Gender was not significantly associated with receipt of prophylaxis: The odds ratio was .81. However, before concluding that the study showed that gender was not important, one must note that the 95% confidence intervals for gender were .06 to 10.12. In other words, it is equally likely that women are a sixteenth as likely or ten times more likely to receive prophylaxis. Obviously, this result is of little scientific value. The study only had 7 women (2% of sample); the model had little information on which to base an estimate of the likelihood of having received prophylaxis for this group and this is reflected in a large standard error and a broad confidence interval. A similar situation can be seen for the variable sexual orientation. Because there were only 31 heterosexuals (10% of sample), the confidence intervals for the risk estimate associated with sexual orientation were very broad: 0.78 to 13.03.

In general, large standard errors and large confidence intervals (which are based on standard errors) are clues of an inadequate sample size. Another, more dramatic indication that you do not have a large enough sample size in logistic regression and proportional hazards analysis is if the model does not converge. There is simply not enough information, usually because of too few outcomes, for the computer to solve the equation. Although you can increase the number of attempts

✓ **T I P**

For multiple linear regression you should have twenty subjects for each independent variable in your model.

[42] Schwarcz, S.K., Katz, M.H., Hirozawa, A., Gurley, R.J., Lemp, G.F. "Prevention of *Pneumocystis carinii* pneumonia: Who are we missing?" *AIDS* 1997; 11:1263–8.

TABLE 7.1

Frequency of primary PCP prophylaxis among patients whose AIDS-defining diagnosis was PCP.

Characteristic	Did not receive PCP prophylaxis n (%)	Received primary PCP prophylaxis n (%)	Adjusted P value	Adjusted odds ratio	95% confidence limits
Total	212 (65.0)	114 (35.0)			
Age group					
<35 years	61 (69.3)	27 (30.7)		1.0 (ref.)	
≥35 years	151 (63.5)	87 (36.6)	0.55	1.19	0.68, 2.07
Ethnicity					
Nonwhite	74 (77.9)	21 (22.1)		0.49	0.28, 0.87
White	138 (59.7)	93 (40.3)	0.01	1.0 (ref.)	
Sex					
Male	206 (64.6)	113 (35.4)		0.81	0.06, 10.12
Female	6 (85.7)	1 (14.3)	0.87	1.0 (ref.)	
Sexual orientation					
Gay/bisexual man	185 (62.7)	110 (37.3)		3.19	0.78, 13.03
Heterosexual	27 (87.1)	4 (12.9)	0.11	1.0 (ref.)	
Injection drug use					
Yes	35 (72.9)	13 (27.1)		1.11	0.49, 2.54
No	177 (63.7)	101 (36.3)	0.80	1.0 (ref.)	
Insurance					
None	52 (82.5)	11 (17.5)		0.35	0.17, 0.73
Public/private	151 (59.5)	103 (40.6)	0.005	1.0 (ref.)	

Adapted with permission from Schwarcz, S.K., et al. "Prevention of *Pneumocystis carinii* pneumonia: Who are we missing?" *AIDS* 1997; 11:1263–8. Copyright Rapid Science Publishers Ltd.

the computer makes to solve the equation (see Section 8.13) if your model fails to converge, you should consider the possibility that you do not have enough subjects to answer your research question.

With multiple linear regression, sample size is not as much an issue as with logistic regression or proportional hazards regression. The reason is that you can consider all subjects as having experienced the outcome (because the outcome is interval). However, just as with these other techniques you will have very large standard errors (and therefore large confidence intervals) if you do not have a large enough sample size. For multiple linear regression twenty subjects (rather than outcome events) per independent variable is recommended.[43] Although this is a very reasonable standard, it does not mean that all analyses with fewer subjects are invalid; you just need to show more caution in interpreting the coefficients.

7.2   What if I have too many independent variables given my sample size?

> ✓ **T I P**
>
> To decide which, if any, variable to eliminate from your analysis, consider theory, measurement, and empirical findings.

If your power calculations or analyses show you have too many independent variables for your sample size, you need to increase the number of subjects or decrease the number of independent variables. Although increasing the number of subjects is more desirable, it is usually impossible in the analysis phase. Most researchers will therefore attempt to reduce the number of independent variables in their analysis. Possible methods are shown in Table 7.2.

7.2.A   Omitting variables

Although you would never want to omit an important variable from your analysis, some variables can be omitted without jeopardizing your analysis. In deciding which, if any, variable to eliminate, consider theory, measurement, and empirical findings.

7.2.A.1   Theoretical considerations for omitting variables.   In the course of your analysis, you may realize that some of the potential independent variables in your data set are not important to your theory or inconsistent with the pathophysiology of the disease you are investigating. For example, in a study of the causes of coronary artery disease, you may have information on whether individuals wore seat belts when driving. In fact, it is even possible that wearing a seat belt is significantly associated with decreased likelihood of coronary artery disease (if seat belt wearers are more health conscious and more likely to follow other health advice, such as having a low fat diet, exercising, etc.). But clearly, wearing seat belts cannot cause or prevent coronary artery disease. Therefore, there is no reason to include it in an analysis of risk factors for coronary artery disease.

---

[43] Feinstein, A.R. *Multivariable Analysis: An Introduction.* New Haven: Yale University Press, 1996, p. 226.

SETTING UP A MULTIVARIABLE ANALYSIS: SUBJECTS

TABLE 7.2
Methods for decreasing the number of independent variables.

---

1. Omitting variables

    Theoretical considerations

    Measurement considerations

        Two variables highly correlated. Omit the one with:

            Larger amount of missing data

            Greater measurement error

            Theoretically less important

    Empirical findings

        Variable unrelated to outcome in bivariate analysis

        Variable unrelated to outcome in multivariable analysis

        Variable unrelated to main independent variable and outcome in bivariate analysis

        Variable has minimal impact on main effect in multivariable analysis

2. Combine variables into a single variable or scale

    "And/or" constructions

    Summation scales

    Factor analysis

7.2.A.2   Measurement considerations for omitting variables   If you have two variables that are moderately correlated with one another, you may want to eliminate one of them. When variables are correlated, by including one, you include some of the information from the other variable. However, unless they are perfectly correlated, you will lose some potentially important information. The amount of information lost depends on the degree of correlation. We have already discussed the issue of variables that are highly or perfectly correlated in the section on multicollinearity (Sections 6.1–6.3). The difference here is that you would be eliminating one of a pair of correlated variables, not because they threaten the validity of your model, but because your sample size is not sufficient to accommodate all your independent variables. In terms of the decision as to which variable to keep and which to exclude, the decision-making process is the same as with multicollinearity. Keep the variable that is theoretically superior, has less missing data, or has lower measurement error.

7.2.A.3 Empirical considerations for omitting variables. You can also decide which variables to exclude based on empirical findings. One common empirical method is to review the bivariate analysis and include only those independent variables that are statistically associated with the outcome. Unless your sample size is very large, it is better to choose a cutoff of what constitutes association that is higher than the standard P value of $<.05$ for determining statistical significance, because weakly associated variables may still be confounders of the main effect. However, variables that are not at all associated with outcome are unlikely to affect your model. Commonly, researchers will include in multivariable models only those independent variables associated with outcomes in bivariate analysis at $P < .15$ or $<.20$. Keep in mind that if you have a suppresser effect, the variable may not be even weakly associated with the outcome in bivariate analysis. (Recall the example in Section 1.3 of zidovudine treatment, which affected the likelihood of seroconversion in multivariable analysis even though it was not significantly related to seroconversion in bivariate analysis.)

Variable selection procedures (statistical algorithms used to select which of your independent variables to include or keep in your multivariable model) can also help you to deal with small sample sizes. These procedures are discussed in Section 8.9.

When you are primarily interested in the association between one main independent variable (e.g., treatment group assignment) and an outcome, you may want to include only those variables that are associated with both the independent variable of interest and the outcome variable in bivariate analyses. Remember, unless both of these conditions are met, the variable cannot be a confounder or suppresser.

A variation of this strategy is to include only those independent variables that change the size of your main effect. For example, Chambers and colleagues studied whether fluoxetine (Prozac) affected birth outcomes.[44] They compared the rate of prematurity among 98 infants whose mothers had taken fluoxetine early in pregnancy only to 70 infants whose mothers had taken it late in pregnancy. Only 14 infants were born prematurely. To limit the number of variables in the model, they included only those independent variables that changed the estimate of the main effect (early only versus late exposure to fluoxetine on prematurity) by more than 10 percent. Eleven variables fit this criterion and were included in the model, in addition to two other

---

[44] Chambers, C.D., Johnson, K.A., Dick, L.M., et al. "Birth outcomes in pregnant women taking fluoxetine." *New Engl. J. Med.* 1996; 335:1010–15.

variables (maternal age and dose of fluoxetine), which were included for theoretical reasons.

With a total of 13 independent variables and only 14 outcomes the investigators were far from fulfilling the guideline of 10 outcomes per variable. Late exposure to fluoxetine was associated with an increased risk of prematurity: odds ratio of 4.8. Reflecting the relatively small number of outcomes and the large number of independent variables, the 95% confidence intervals for the effect of fluoxetine on prematurity were large, ranging from 1.1 to 20.8. Because the confidence intervals excluded 1, the data suggest that late exposure to fluoxetine is associated with an increased risk of prematurity. However, in weighing the benefits versus risks, there is a large difference between an odds ratio of 1.1 and one of 20.8.

7.2.B Methods of combining variables into a single variable or scale

Sometimes you can reduce the number of independent variables in your analysis without omitting a variable. This is done by combining variables into a single variable or scale. Three methods are commonly used: "and/or" constructions, summation scales, and factor analysis.

7.2.B.1 Use of "and/or" constructions. Two or more related variables can be combined with the use of an "and/or" clause (Section 6.3). For example, in the study of the effect of perinatal exposure to fluoxetine on birth outcomes, the investigators combined hypertension, preeclampsia, and eclampsia as one variable. In other words, women who suffered from hypertension, preeclampsia, eclampsia, or more than one of the three, would be "yes" on the variable; women who had none of these conditions would be "no". This fits the pathophysiology in that the three conditions are progressive states of the same underlying condition. And/or clauses may also be helpful when you have variables that are multicollinear (all women with eclampsia by definition have preeclampsia) or when you have an independent variable with almost everyone in the same group (as you would if you had a variable eclampsia yes/no – almost everyone would be no, since eclampsia is relatively rare). Independent variables where almost everyone is in the same group tend to have large standard errors and large confidence intervals.

7.2.B.2 Summation scales. Investigators may use scales (sets of closely related questions) to measure constructs that are difficult to assess by a single question (e.g., functional status, attitudes). The decision to create a scale is usually made in the design phase, although researchers sometimes find, in the analytic phase, that a group of variables measure a reliable construct.

To summate a scale, first code all questions in the same direction, so that, for example, a higher score is better on all items. You must also recode variables so that they are all on the same numeric scales. Otherwise variables measured on a 0 to 10 scale will have twice the weight in the total score as variables measured on a 0 to 5 scale. Dividing a 0 to 10 scale by two will put it on the same scale as a 0 to 5 scale. Once you summate the variables, if you then divide the scale by the number of variables in the scale, a subject's value will equal the average of their responses to the variables that constitute the scale.

In creating scales you must pay close attention to the handling of missing data on individual items. If, for a particular subject, the majority of items that constitute the scale have missing values then the value for the scale should be missing for that subject. If at least half of the items, for a particular subject, have a valid response, you can replace the missing value with the mean for the sample on the particular item. Once you have replaced the missing values, you can then summate the scale and divide by the number of variables in the scale.

There is an alternative method for handling missing cases when constructing scales. You can compute the average for each subject by dividing by the number of variables for which the subject has valid responses. For example, if a particular subject had valid responses for four of the five variables that constitute a scale, you could summate their four questions and divide by four. In comparison, for subjects with complete values, you would summate their five questions and divide by five. If you are using this technique, at least half of the variables that constitute the scale for each subject must have complete data. Assign a missing value to subjects who have more than half the variables with missing data. (Some would assign a missing value if a fourth or more of the questions have missing responses.)[45]

These types of summations will work only if the variables are highly correlated. The usual measure of how correlated the variables are to one another is the alpha (also referred to as a reliability coefficient). Alphas greater than 0.65 generally indicate that the variables

[45] Hull, C.H., Nie, N.H. *SPSS Update 7–9*. New York: McGraw-Hill, 1989, p. 257.

form a reliable scale. To achieve alphas of this level, the questions are usually written with the intention of scoring them together.

Factor analysis is a popular strategy in the behavioral sciences for reducing the number of variables in cases where you have multiple related independent variables. Factor analysis summarizes multiple related independent variables (say 15) into a few underlying factors (say 2 or 3). The procedure minimizes the correlations between the factors (so that they truly represent distinct dimensions). Each factor is a weighted combination of the original variables. As such you can develop a factor score for each subject based on that subject's values for each of the variables, thereby reducing the number of variables to the number of factors. Each of the independent variables will be correlated with each of the factors, but to varying degrees. For any one of the factors, a few of the variables will be strongly correlated with it, indicating that the factor primarily represents this cluster of variables. Based on these correlations (referred to as loadings) you can characterize the nature of the factor (i.e., what it represents).

The major problem with factor analysis for clinical researchers is the loss of the original variables. Let's say, for example, you used factor analysis to develop factor scores for variables associated with survival with pneumonia. Assume the first factor was characterized by patient comorbidity (age, underlying lung disease, history of congestive heart failure), the second factor was characterized by virulence of attack (severity of radiological findings, peak of fever, specific organism recovered), and the third factor was characterized by efficacy of treatment (speed of first dose, appropriate choice of antibiotics). This would be a very satisfying summation of the data from the point of view of the pathophysiology of pneumonia.

Assume that a proportional hazards model demonstrates that the factors patient comorbidity and virulence of attack are associated with a worse survival, whereas efficacious treatment is associated with an improved survival. How useful would these results be to a clinician? Certainly, clinicians could not use the information to generate a probability of survival for their patients because it would be mathematically too complicated to generate factor scores. Also, you couldn't tell clinicians how important any one variable was to the outcome (only the importance of the factor to the outcome). Whereas a particular variable may have a strong loading on a factor that is related to outcome, that variable may be only weakly related to outcome. This is because factor analysis groups independent variables based on their

> **DEFINITION**
>
> *Factor analysis* summarizes multiple related independent variables (say 15) into a few underlying factors (say 2 or 3).

> ✓ **TIP**
>
> The major problem with factor analysis for clinical researchers is the loss of the original variables.

relationship to one another, not their relationship to the outcome variable.

For these reasons, factor analysis has a relatively small place in the analysis of medically oriented data. In the behavioral sciences, where we are dealing with constructs that are complicated to measure (e.g., self-esteem, autonomy) the "loss" of single variables is more than compensated for by the strength of the technique for dealing with multiple related independent variables.[46]

7.3 What if some of my subjects do not complete my study?

It is common in longitudinal clinical studies for subjects to not complete the study. There are a variety of reasons for this. Subjects may decide they no longer wish to participate. They may move. They may die. They may have to be withdrawn due to a side effect they have developed. Sometimes you will not know why the person is lost to follow-up; they just are.

Coping with subjects who do not finish a study is one major way in which clinical research is different from other types of research. In laboratory research, it is usually possible to control conditions (e.g., laboratory animals, cell cultures) so that no observations are lost. Much of social science research (and some clinical research) is conducted using cross-sectional designs (surveying people about independent variables and outcomes at the same time). Thus while there are always people who choose not to participate, subjects are not lost during the study. However, for longitudinal studies (studies of people over time) we need a way to deal with persons who do not complete the study.

One method of dealing with such subjects is to delete them. However, in a long study you may eventually lose a substantial portion of your initial sample. Also, people who have participated for, say, three or four years of a five year study have vital information to contribute. Finally, you introduce bias into your study when you delete subjects. What we would ideally like is a technique that allows subjects to contribute information until they leave the study. Such a technique exists. It is called censoring and it is a major element of all types of survival analysis, including proportional hazards analysis.

----

[46] For more on factor analysis see: Glantz, S.A., Slinker, B.K. *Primer of Applied Regression and Analysis of Variance*. New York: McGraw-Hill, 1990, pp. 216–36; Kleinbaum, D.G., Kupper, L.L., Muller, K.E. *Applied Regression Analysis and Other Multivariable Methods* (2nd ed.). Boston: PWS-Kent, 1988, pp. 595–640.

Coping with subjects who do not finish a study is one major way in which clinical research is different from other types of research.

Censoring allows subjects to contribute information until they leave the study.

All subjects in a proportional hazards analysis who do not experience the outcome of interest are censored, if not during the course of the study, then at the end of the study.

SETTING UP A MULTIVARIABLE ANALYSIS: SUBJECTS

TABLE 7.3
Reasons for censoring observations.

Reason for censoring	Examples
1. Lost to follow-up.	Subject moves, doesn't wish to participate, stops attending a particular clinic.
2. Subject has an outcome that precludes the outcome you are studying: (also known as alternative outcomes or competing risks.)	Death from coronary artery disease in a study of cancer incidence.
3. Subject is withdrawn from study.	Development of side effects, not ethical to continue treatment or placebo.
4. Varying dates of enrollment.	Study enrolls subjects with different starting dates over a 2-year period.
5. End of study.	All subjects who have not experienced outcome are considered censored at the end of the study.

Besides allowing us to incorporate subjects who are lost to follow-up, censoring has broader implications. It allows us to analyze, within one study, subjects with unequal lengths of follow-up for a variety of reasons (Table 7.3). Indeed, all subjects in a proportional hazards analysis who do not experience the outcome of interest are censored, if not during the course of the study, then at the end of the study.

7.4 What assumptions does censoring make about observations with unequal lengths of follow-up?

Censoring assumes that if subjects could be followed beyond the point in time when they are censored, they would have the same rate of outcome as those not censored at that time. Another way of saying this is that the censoring occurs randomly, independent of outcome.

To understand the principles of censoring, let's look at a Kaplan–Meier survival graph of 100 persons shown in Figure 7.1. The tick marks on the survival function show where persons are censored, that is, leave the analysis. Under the *x* axis of Figure 7.1, I have shown the number of persons who are at risk for outcome (i.e., have not yet experienced the outcome and have not been censored) and the percent survival.

> Censoring assumes that if subjects could be followed beyond the point in time when they are censored, they would have the same rate of outcome as those not censored at that time.

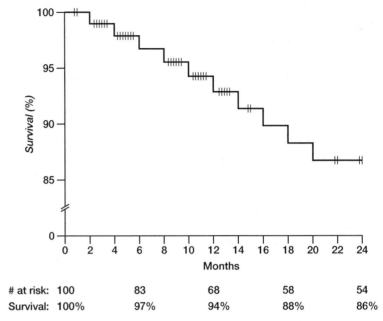

| # at risk: | 100 | 83 | 68 | 58 | 54 |
| Survival: | 100% | 97% | 94% | 88% | 86% |

Figure 7.1. Hypothetical survival experience of 100 subjects.

At time 0, everyone is alive and we have 100% survival. As time passes, people die and percent survival decreases. At two years, survival is 86%. Does this mean that 14 participants died and 86 are still alive? No. In fact, there were only 10 deaths.

When you have censoring, the probability of surviving to the end of the follow-up period is not simply the proportion of the original sample known to be alive at the end of the study. The censored subjects contribute information only until the time that they leave the analysis. To account for this, we compute a current event rate based on the number of subjects alive and not censored at each point that an event occurs. These current event rates can then be used to compute cumulative survival at the end of the study period (in this case two years). Here's how.

Survival to the end is equivalent to surviving each moment in the entire period. We can write the probability of surviving each moment as a product: the product of surviving the first moment times the conditional probability of surviving the second, given that you survived the first, times the conditional probability of surviving the third, given that you survived the first two, and so on, through the last moment.

SETTING UP A MULTIVARIABLE ANALYSIS: SUBJECTS

In turn, we can estimate each of these conditional probabilities as one minus the current event rate.

The cumulative survival at a particular time is simply the conditional probability for that time multiplied by the conditional probability for the prior time at which an event occurred. Because the conditional probabilities are multiplied, this method is sometimes referred to as the product-limit method. For all moments when no event occurs (such as at three months in Figure 7.1 and Table 7.4 when there are six censored subjects but no outcome events), the conditional probability is one, and so it doesn't change the product. These calculations are illustrated in Table 7.4.

Note that censored observations contribute to the analysis until they leave the study, with the provision that they must be in the study at the time that at least one outcome event occurs. Looked at from a different perspective, if observations are censored before any events occur, as is the case with the two censored observations that occur in this example at one month, the censored observations would not contribute to the analysis at all (because to be included in the denominator of the current event rate they must still be in the study when the outcome occurs.)

What does survival analysis assume about those persons who are censored? It assumes that they would have the same survival experience as those who stayed in the analysis. So if all subjects could be followed to two years in my hypothetical example, how many would have died? The answer is 14. Why? Because, if no one were censored, then at two years, we would have the full sample size of 100. To yield a survival rate of 86%, 14 persons would have died.

I'm sure you can appreciate that this is not an insignificant assumption you are making about censored observations. After all, you can not prove that censored observations have the same survival experience as those uncensored. If you actually knew the time to outcome for the censored observations they wouldn't need to be censored. What you as an investigator must address is the likelihood that the censoring assumption is valid based on your understanding of why people have been censored (Section 7.5).

Although I have put both tick marks on the survival curve and put the number of subjects at risk for outcome under the graph, most published studies will show you one or the other. The number of persons at risk decreases as persons are censored or experience the outcome.

TABLE 7.4

Calculation of cumulative survival.

Study time (months)	# of subjects at risk for outcome	# of outcomes	# censored	Current event rate(# outcomes/ # subject at risk)	Conditional probability (1−current event rate)	Cumulative survival
1	100	0	2	$0/100 = 0$	$1 - 0 = 1$	1
2	98	1	0	$1/98 = .01$	$1 - .01 = .99$	$(1)(.99) = .99$
3	97	0	6	$0/97 = 0$	$1 - 0 = 1$	$(.99)(1) = .99$
4	91	1	0	$1/91 = .01$	$1 - .01 = .99$	$(.99)(.99) = .98$
5	90	0	7	$0/90 = 0$	$1 - 0 = 1$	$(.98)(1) = .98$
6	83	1	0	$1/83 = .01$	$1 - .01 = .99$	$(.98)(.99) = .97$
8	82	1	0	$1/82 = .01$	$1 - .01 = .99$	$(.97)(.99) = .96$
9	81	0	6	$0/81 = 0$	$1 - 0 = 1$	$(.96)(1) = .96$
10	75	1	0	$1/75 = .01$	$1 - .01 = .99$	$(.96)(.99) = .95$
11	74	0	6	$0/74 = 0$	$1 - 0 = 1$	$(.95)(1) = .95$
12	68	1	0	$1/68 = .01$	$1 - .01 = .99$	$(.95)(.99) = .94$
13	67	0	5	$0/67 = 0$	$1 - 0 = 1$	$(.94)(1) = .94$
14	62	1	0	$1/62 = .02$	$1 - .02 = .98$	$(.94)(.98) = .92$
15	61	0	2	$0/61 = 0$	$1 - 0 = 1$	$(.92)(1) = .92$
16	59	1	0	$1/59 = .02$	$1 - .02 = .98$	$(.92)(.98) = .90$
18	58	1	0	$1/58 = .02$	$1 - .02 = .98$	$(.90)(.98) = .88$
20	57	1	0	$1/57 = .02$	$1 - .02 = .98$	$(.88)(.98) = .86$
22	56	0	2	$0/56 = 0$	$1 - 0 = 1$	$(.86)(1) = .86$
24	54	0	2	$0/54 = 0$	$1 - 0 = 1$	$(.86)(1) = .86$

Sometimes published survival curves do not show either ticks for censored observations or the number of subjects at risk as the study progresses. This is a serious limitation because without this information you cannot assess how much the sample is shrinking as the study progresses. As the sample shrinks, the data no longer represent the survival experience of the full sample. One tip-off that there may be a problem is if the curve begins to have large "steps." As the sample size decreases, the steps of the curve become larger, because an outcome makes a larger difference in the proportion surviving. This is illustrated in Figure 7.1 and Table 7.4. (Note in the table that a single outcome occurring at the end of the study has a larger current event rate than an outcome occurring earlier on in the study.)

7.5 How likely is it that the censoring assumption is valid in my study?

The likelihood that the censoring assumption is valid depends a great deal on the reason for the censored observations.

7.5.A Loss to follow-up

Subjects may be lost to follow-up because they have grown weary of participating in a study (especially if it involves frequent office visits and blood draws). Loss to follow-up is especially common in retrospective medical record review studies. From the medical record you may not know what has happened to the subject. You will know only that after a certain period of time there were no further entries into the chart.

Of all reasons for censoring, losses to follow-up are the most problematic for meeting the censoring assumptions. Since the participants are lost, you are unlikely to know what has happened to them after leaving the study. For this reason, assuming that the rate of outcome for the censored observations is the same as that for the uncensored subjects may be problematic. Also, several studies have found that persons who drop out of studies are different from those who remain in the study. For example, a randomized controlled trial of zidovudine in HIV-infected persons found that persons who were lost to follow-up were more likely to have deteriorating immune function during the trial than those who remained in the trial.[47] (They probably left the trial because they knew they were not doing well and wanted to seek other treatment.)

> Of all reasons for censoring, losses to follow-up are the most problematic for meeting the censoring assumptions.

7.5.B Alternative outcome

Some of your subjects may need to be censored because they experience an outcome that precludes the outcome of interest in your study. This is often referred to as competing risks. For example, consider a

---

[47] Volberding, P.A., Lagakos, S.W., Koch, M.A., et al. "Zidovudine in asymptomatic human immunodeficiency virus infection: A controlled trial in persons with fewer than 500 CD4-positive cells per cubic millimeter." *N. Engl. J. Med.* 1990; 322:941–9.

study that randomized persons with atrial fibrillation to warfarin or to standard of care treatment at that time (aspirin or no treatment at all).[48] Stroke was the outcome of interest. The investigators therefore censored persons who died from causes other than stroke (e.g., cardiac events, cancer).

Although it is common to censor persons who have an alternative outcome that precludes the outcome of interest, most studies with a main outcome other than death will also report the results for death as an outcome. There are several reasons for this. Even if warfarin prevents stroke in patients with atrial fibrillation as shown in this study, if subjects treated with warfarin do not also live longer, the therapy may not be as strongly recommended. Your view of warfarin as a treatment certainly would be swayed by knowing that the rate of stroke was lower but the rate of death was higher. This could happen if the treatment was effective against stroke but had a life-threatening side effect.

Another reason to include death as an outcome is that there may be some question as to whether an alternative outcome truly excludes the outcome of interest. Even events that appear unrelated to the outcome of interest may be related. In the context of the atrial fibrillation study, consider someone who died in a car accident. Could you be certain that they did not have a stroke while behind the wheel?

To minimize bias in determining whether an outcome is truly unrelated to the outcome of interest, a study should have objective a priori criteria as to what constitutes an alternative outcome. In addition, judgments on individual cases should be made by a review committee that is masked to the treatment assignment. This is exactly what was done in the study of warfarin in patients with atrial fibrillation.

However, even with the best criteria and objective reviews, you may mistakenly assume that some outcomes are unrelated to your outcome of interest when, perhaps, they are related. In the atrial fibrillation study there were 37 deaths; only one was due to stroke. The warfarin group had a lower rate of death overall, a lower rate of death due to cardiac causes, and a lower rate of death due to noncardiac causes. Since warfarin was not anticipated to have any effect on mortality other than decreasing deaths due to stroke, these findings suggest

✓ **TIP**

To minimize bias in determining whether an outcome is truly unrelated to the outcome of interest, a study should have objective a priori criteria as to what constitutes an alternative outcome.

---

[48] The Boston Area Anticoagulation Trial for Atrial Fibrillation Investigators. "The effect of low-dose warfarin on the risk of stroke in patients with nonrheumatic atrial fibrillation." *N. Engl. J. Med.* 1990; 323:1505–11.

SETTING UP A MULTIVARIABLE ANALYSIS: SUBJECTS

two possibilities. Warfarin may prevent death due to other causes or some of the deaths due to other causes may have actually been due to unrecognized strokes. The possibility of unrecognized strokes does not weaken the findings. If there were missed strokes in the nonwarfarin group it would only strengthen the treatment effect of warfarin. But for the purposes of this discussion, I think this is a good example of how hard it is to correctly categorize nonoutcome related events.

When death is a common alternative outcome, as it is in any long-term study of elderly or very ill people, competing mortality may bias your estimates of time to outcome. This will occur if the likelihood of outcome would have been higher in those persons who died had they not died. The bias of competing risks can be avoided by not using outcomes other than death (since no outcome precludes death). But in many cases we are interested in these other outcomes. A reasonable compromise is to report both (as was done in the atrial fibrillation trial). More sophisticated methods for dealing with competing risks are beyond the scope of this book.[49]

> When death is a common alternative outcome, competing mortality may bias your estimates of time to outcome.

7.5.C Withdrawal

Persons may withdraw from a study because they do not think the treatment is helping, because they want to receive a treatment and believe they were randomized to placebo, because they have a side effect, or because they find the protocol too demanding of their time. Subjects are usually withdrawn by the investigators for safety reasons (a side effect that makes it dangerous for the subject to continue treatment).

Less commonly, investigators may withdraw a subject because they develop a condition that precludes them from participating in one of the arms of the study. For example, in the study of warfarin in atrial fibrillation, the investigators had to withdraw a participant who required valvular replacement during the study. Why? Although valvular replacement does not preclude the development of stroke nor is it a side effect of treatment (or nontreatment), a patient receiving valvular replacement requires anticoagulation with warfarin. Since treatment with warfarin was mandatory, the person could not be continued in a study comparing warfarin to standard treatment.

---

[49] Pepe, M.S., Longton, G., Pettinger, M., Mori, M., Fisher, D.L., Storb, R. "Summarizing data on survival, relapse, and chronic graft-versus-host disease after bone marrow transplantation: Motivation for and description of new methods." *Br. J. Haematol.* 1993; 83:602–7.

At first glance, subjects who voluntarily withdraw or are withdrawn by the investigators may seem like losses to follow-up, but there is an important difference. The difference is that withdrawn participants may be willing to let you passively follow them for outcome, even though they do not want to actively participate in your protocol. (This may not be true if they have a side effect and blame you for it!) If the withdrawn subjects will allow you to follow them for outcome, you do not have to censor them prior to the end of the study. Instead you can perform an intention-to-treat analysis.

Intention-to-treat means that participants are counted as members of their originally assigned group, no matter what happens during the study period. For example, in a study with a treatment and a placebo arm, if you perform an intention-to-treat analysis, persons who were assigned to treatment would be part of the treatment group even if they stopped taking the treatment during the study. Intention-to-treat analysis protects against treatments appearing to be more favorable than they are. If subjects with side effects are less likely to benefit from treatment than those without side effects, removing them from the analysis at the time of their side effect will bias your results. It will make your treatment appear more effective than it is. For example, if 100 people are given a new treatment that is effective but causes nausea so severe that only 50% of subjects are able to tolerate the treatment long enough to benefit from it, removing 50 study participants will make the treatment look more effective than it is (because a very high proportion of those subjects left in the trial will benefit from the treatment).

The downside of intention-to-treat analysis is that it dilutes the effect of treatment. Keeping to the same example, if you keep 50 subjects who did not take the full treatment in your treatment arm, the treatment arm will be similar to the nontreatment arm. You might ask: Isn't this justified? What good is a treatment if patients can not tolerate it? But remember there is a difference between a sample and an individual patient. If I had a terrible disease, I might be interested in trying an efficacious medicine that caused unrelenting vomiting for 50% of persons. After all, if I am in the half of persons who doesn't develop vomiting, why should I forgo an efficacious treatment? If the authors only report the results of the intention-to-treat analysis you would not know how efficacious the treatment is for the subgroup of people who can tolerate it. Limiting your analysis to persons who tolerate or comply with treatment is sometimes referred to as an efficacy analysis (how efficacious is the treatment for people who take it) whereas intention-to-treat analysis is referred to as an effectiveness analysis (how effective is the treatment in the real world).

If the number of subjects who stop treatment or withdraw from your study is small, it won't matter whether you perform intention-to-treat analysis or censor them at the time they leave the study. Since intention-to-treat is a more conservative approach for estimating the efficacy of treatment than censoring subjects when they withdraw from a treatment arm, most researchers prefer it. In studies where a large number of subjects are withdrawn, you may want to report the analysis both ways.

7.5.D Varying time of enrollment

Varying times of enrollment (starting times) is an important issue for large prospective studies and for studies of rare diseases. For studies enrolling thousands of participants, logistic constraints preclude everyone from starting the study on the same day. Most large studies are conducted in multiple centers and it is rare for all sites to begin enrollment at the same time. Similarly, with studies of rare diseases it may take several years to identify and enroll enough persons.

In observational studies, varying times of enrollment is the rule, rather than the exception. For example, in the Aerobics Center Longitudinal Study discussed in Section 1.1, the investigators enrolled participants over a nineteen-year period. Indeed, their study is an open cohort with ongoing accrual of subjects. Subjects are enrolled when they complete the baseline medical examination and are then followed prospectively. Similarly, the study of survival with melanoma, discussed in Section 2.1C, followed patients diagnosed over a nine-year period.

Theoretically, varying start times could be dealt with by following all subjects for a fixed time period (e.g., three years) regardless of when they started the study. In this instance, no one will be censored prior to the end of the study due to varying lengths of enrollment. However, this method would decrease the power of the analysis because you would lose the additional follow-up time supplied by the persons who began the study early on. In most studies, the greatest cost (in time and funds) is the initial enrollment and evaluation. The cost of continuing follow-up for the outcome is usually minimal, while the gain, in terms of follow-up time, can be great. Also, waiting until the last enrolled participant completes a preset follow-up period will extend the length of the study often beyond the time that the analytic staff is being supported. Finally, we are all impatient to learn the results of our work.

> ✓ **T I P**
>
> Intention-to-treat is a more conservative approach for estimating the efficacy of treatment than censoring subjects when they withdraw from one of the treatment arms.

Thus, most investigators will censor results at a common point in calendar time. At this point in time, length of follow-up will differ for the participants. If the longest follow-up is three years, all participants who have follow-up less than three years and have not experienced an outcome will be censored at the amount of time of follow-up, which in all cases will be less than three years. Those with three years of follow-up and no outcome will be censored at three years.

7.5.E End of study

It may have surprised you that a subject who completes a study (or who in an observational trial has the longest follow-up) without experiencing the outcome still is censored. This is counter intuitive because in common usage we think of censored subjects as those that do not complete the study. Although all subjects who do not experience the study outcome are ultimately censored, there is an important difference between those censored at the end of a trial and those censored for other reasons. The difference is that for those subjects censored at the end of the study, no assumptions need be made about the future – the study is over. Usually, in the published report, the authors will tell you the date that subjects who completed the study without experiencing an outcome were censored. It is the last date of the study or the last day of observation.

7.6 How can I test the validity of the censoring assumption for my data?

There is no ideal test for assessing the validity of the censoring assumption. It is primarily a judgment call by the investigators, reviewers, and readers of the data. That's why in Section 7.5 I took you through a long discussion of the reasons for censoring and how censored observations may or may not fulfill the assumptions of censoring. Nonetheless, it is possible to make a general assessment about censored observations. First, and foremost, studies that have a large number of censored observations prior to the end of the study are more problematic than studies that have just a few censored observations.

Graphical methods, showing when during the trial censoring occurred, provide a test of the validity of the censoring assumption. Figures 7.2a and 7.2b show two very different patterns of censoring. In Figure 7.2a it would appear that subjects (shown with asterisks) dropped out evenly through the course of the study. In Figure 7.2b it would appear that a clump of subjects dropped out around six months.

> **✓ TIP**
>
> Studies that have a large number of censored observations prior to the end of the study are more problematic than studies that have just a few censored observations.

> **✓ TIP**
>
> Censored observations occurring evenly throughout the study are consistent with the censoring assumption whereas clumps of censored observations suggest nonrandom censoring.

SETTING UP A MULTIVARIABLE ANALYSIS: SUBJECTS

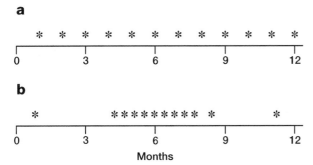

Figure 7.2. Different patterns of censoring. In Figure 7.2a censored observations have occurred evenly over the study period whereas in Figure 7.2b censored observations are clumped at 6 months.

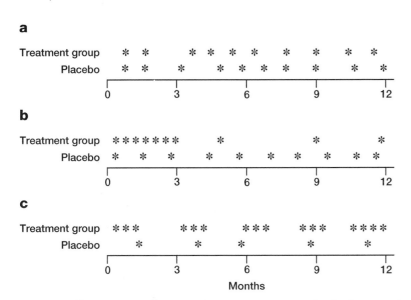

Figure 7.3. Different patterns of censoring between a treatment and a placebo group. In Figure 7.3a the patterns of censoring between the two groups are similar. In Figure 7.3b there are an equal number of censored observations in the two groups, but the pattern is different. In Figure 7.3c, there are more censored observations in the treatment group than in the placebo group.

Whereas the latter suggests some event that occurred at around six months, the former suggests the kind of censoring that you would expect if people dropped out for random reasons such as moving out of town, other obligations, etc.

Graphical displays can also be used to compare censoring in two or more different arms of a study. Figures 7.3a–c show a treatment and a placebo group. Note how in Figure 7.3a the number of persons censored between the treatment and placebo groups is the same and the pattern of censoring between the two groups is also similar. In Figure 7.3b, the number of censored persons is the same but the pattern between the two groups is different. In Figure 7.3c, there are many more censored observations in the treatment group. Whereas Figure 7.3a is consistent with random censoring, Figures 7.3b and 7.3c suggest that the causes of censored observations are different for the treatment and placebo group.

Besides graphical models, there are other methods for assessing the validity of the censoring assumption. You can answer the question of whether subjects lost to follow-up are different from those not lost to follow-up by modeling who is most likely to be lost to follow-up. This can be based on baseline characteristics. So, for example, you can examine whether there are differences by age, race, etc. of persons lost to follow-up compared to persons not lost to follow-up. In particular, you might wish to explore whether subjects at high risk of outcome are differentially lost to follow-up. The censoring assumption can also be tested using time-dependent covariates (Sections 12.4 and 12.5)

To be certain that censoring due to alternative outcomes is not affecting your results, report rate of death where possible, in addition to whatever more proximal outcome you are studying. Since there is no alternative outcome to death (no alternative outcome can exclude death), these curves reassure the reader.

For withdrawn cases, it is best to test the censoring assumption by conducting intention-to-treat analyses as described above. Since you can continue to follow withdrawn patients for outcome, you can test whether leaving them in or taking them out makes a difference.

Censoring due to varying starting times is usually assumed to fulfill the censoring assumptions since subjects who enroll at the start of a study should be the same as subjects who enroll in the end. I say "should be," because sometimes investigators become more flexible about the enrollment criteria as studies progress, especially if enrollment is running slowly. Changing the enrollment criteria after a study has begun should be avoided.

But even assuming a group of investigators rigidly used the same enrollment criteria over the course of a long study, one should compare subjects enrolled in the early years of a study to those enrolled in the later years. The reason is that subjects enrolled in later years

SETTING UP A MULTIVARIABLE ANALYSIS: SUBJECTS

may be more likely to have received technical advances that were not available in the earlier years of the study. If they were, and these advances could affect development of the outcome of interest, then the assumptions of censoring are not valid.

In conclusion, censoring is a very helpful tool for clinical research. It prevents you from having to delete valuable cases. A randomized controlled trial comparing fluoride to placebo for the prevention of fractures among women with osteoporosis greatly benefited from censoring.[50] Only 135 (67%) of the 202 enrolled women were able to complete four years of treatment. If the investigators had deleted these cases they would have lost a third of their sample size. As with any powerful statistical tool, however, censoring should be used carefully. Ask yourself (and tell your reader) the circumstances of persons censored. When you know the outcome of censored cases, perform intention-to-treat analyses.

---

[50] Riggs, B.L., Hodgson, S.F., O'Fallon, W.M., et al. "Effect of fluoride treatment on the fracture rate in postmenopausal women with osteoporosis." *N. Engl. J. Med.* 1990; 322:802–9.

8

Performing the Analysis

8.1 What numbers should I assign for dichotomous or ordinal variables in my analysis?

Let's take the simplest case of a dichotomous predictor variable based on an interview question: Do you have a history of diabetes: yes or no?

The equations used to solve multivariable analysis need numerical representations of yes and no. Since this scale only has two points, the numeric distance between the two points can be represented by any two numbers that are separated by one: 0 and 1, 1 and 2, 0 and −1, etc. It doesn't really matter. The sign of the coefficient may change depending on whether you assign "yes" the higher or the lower value, but the coefficient and significance level will be the same (Section 9.3). However, you will not get the same answer if you code your variables such that there is more than one point between the two numbers. For example, coding schemes like +1 and −1 will give you a different answer because there is more than one unit between the two points.

Although any two numbers that are one number apart will give you the same answer, a sensible convention, for both independent and dependent variables, is to use 1 and 0, with 1 representing the presence and 0 representing the absence of the condition. This convention is easy to remember and decreases the chance that you will be confused at the direction of the effect. This coding scheme has another advantage: When a variable is coded this way, the mean of the variable represents the prevalence of the condition. For example, if you have 100 subjects and 10 experience the outcome, the mean of the variable (if coded 0,1) will be $[(0 \times 90) + (1 \times 10)]/100 = .10$. This can be handy when you want to know the prevalence of a risk factor or outcome in a particular group of patients.

> ✓ **TIP**
>
> Code your variables as 1 = presence of condition and 0 = absence of the condition; then the mean of the variable will be equal to the prevalence of the condition.

For some independent variables, such as gender, where there is no absence or presence of a condition, assign the 1 to the value that will make the most sense in how you will discuss your results. For example, if your hypothesis is that women with coronary artery disease receive fewer procedures due to gender bias, it would be sensible to assign women the 1 and men the 0.

8.2 Does it matter what I choose as my reference category for multiple dichotomous ("dummied") variables?

We have reviewed how to create multiple dichotomous variables from a single variable to represent nominal and ordinal variables (Section 4.2) and how to use multiple dichotomous variables to deal with predictor variables that are related to outcome in a nonlinear fashion (Section 5.5).

In Section 4.2 I explained that a variable representing the reference group will not be entered into the analysis; rather the other categories will be compared to this group. Given that, does it matter which category you choose as your reference group? The answer is that your choice of reference group makes a difference in how you report your results and a small difference in the results themselves.

Table 8.1 illustrates the implications of varying your reference group. Assume the data are from a study on the association between ethnicity and access to health care. In column 1, the reference group is

TABLE 8.1
Implications of changing the reference group for dichotomous variables.

	Odds ratio	Odds ratio
White/Caucasian	1.0 (reference)	4.0
African-American	0.25	1.0 (reference)
Latino	0.50	2.0
Asian/Pacific Islander	0.50	2.0
Native American	0.25	1.0
Other nonwhite ethnicity	0.50	2.0

white/Caucasian. The odds ratios indicate that African Americans and Native Americans are a fourth as likely as whites/Caucasians to receive medical care, whereas Latinos, Asian/Pacific Islanders, and other non-whites are half as likely as whites/Caucasians to receive medical care.

Column 2 lists exactly the same data, but now African-Americans are the reference group. We see that whites are still four times more likely to receive medical care as African-Americans. Latinos, Asian/Pacific Islanders, and other nonwhites are about twice as likely as African-Americans to receive medical care, whereas Native Americans are equally likely as African Americans to have received medical care.

Although column 1 and 2 are mathematically equivalent, the reporting of the results is slightly different. If the hypothesis of your study was that persons of color have less access to medical care than persons who are white/Caucasian, it would be sensible to have the white/Caucasian group be the reference group as in column 1. This gives you the ability to report to your readers how access to medical care differs for persons of color compared to persons who are white/Caucasian. If you made African-Americans your reference group as in column 2, you would not be able to directly compare Latino, Asian-Pacific Islanders, Native Americans, and other nonwhites to the white/Caucasian group because the reference is to African-Americans. If, however, your research question concerns whether African-Americans are less or more likely to receive medical care than other ethnicities, coding African-Americans as the reference category, as in column 2, is sensible.

For this reason, investigators generally choose the reference category based on the main hypothesis being tested. If you have no main hypothesis, and your dummied variables represent an interval variable (such as age), it is generally easier to report your results in a manner consistent with your empirical findings. For example, if age is associated with increasing (or decreasing) rate of outcome, you should use the extreme category (e.g., the youngest or the oldest subjects) as the reference group. This allows you to summarize your results by saying older persons are more likely (or less likely) than younger persons (the reference category) to experience the outcome. Conversely if the variable underlying the dummied variables has a **U**-shaped distribution (Section 5.5), it may be best to code the middle group as the reference group so that you can demonstrate the elevated risk at the two extremes.

Which group you choose as your reference group makes a small statistical difference. If you choose the largest group as your reference category, the standard errors will be slightly smaller and the confidence intervals will be somewhat narrower because the model has a larger comparison group and can therefore make more precise estimates. Although this is not a major factor in most studies, if your hypothesis and empirical findings do not lead you to choose a particular category as your reference group, choose the one with the largest sample size.

8.3 How do I enter interaction terms into my analysis?

In Section 1.4 I explained that an interaction occurs when the association of an independent variable on outcome is changed by the value of a third variable. How do you deal with interaction terms in a multivariable analysis?

The most common method of incorporating an interaction in a multivariable model is to create a product term. This is done by creating a variable whose value is the product of two independent variables (i.e., the two variables multiplied by each other). A product term between two independent variables is referred to as a two-way interaction or a primary interaction. A product term between three independent variables is referred to as a three-way interaction or a secondary interaction.

In Section 1.4 I reviewed an example of an interaction between gender and ST elevations. The coding for the product term for male gender and ST elevations is shown in Table 8.2. Note that the two variables male gender (yes/no) and ST elevations (yes/no) divide the sample into four groups: men with ST elevations, men without ST elevations, women with ST elevations, and women without ST elevations. Each cell has its own unique combination of these two variables. In

> ✓ **TIP**
>
> If your hypothesis and empirical findings do not lead you to choose a particular category as your reference group, choose the one with the largest sample size.

> The most common method of incorporating an interaction in a multivariable model is to create a product term.

TABLE 8.2
Creation of an interaction (product) term.

Male gender	ST elevations	
	Yes (= 1)	No (= 0)
Yes (= 1)	$1 \times 1 = \mathbf{1}$	$1 \times 0 = \mathbf{0}$
No (= 0)	$0 \times 1 = \mathbf{0}$	$0 \times 0 = \mathbf{0}$

bold is the value of the product term. Note how the product term highlights those subjects who have both risk factors (male and ST elevations).

To determine if an interaction was present between male gender and ST elevations, the authors entered the product term into their multiple logistic regression analysis, along with the two variables constituting the product term (male gender and ST elevations). If there had been no interaction, meaning the effect of the two risk factors on outcome (heart attack) is captured by the two variables, male gender and ST elevations, then the product term would have been nonsignificant. The authors would have established that there was no interaction between male gender and ST elevations. Instead the product term was significant indicating that there was an interaction. In this case the sign on the product term was negative, indicating that the effect of being male and having ST elevations had significantly less impact on the likelihood of heart attack then you would have expected from the individual effects of male gender and hypertension.

Because a product term describes the relationship between two risk factors and an outcome, it can only be interpreted as an interaction if the two risk factors (in this case male gender and ST elevations) are in the model. If you enter only the product term, without assessing the individual risk factors in the model and the product term is significant, you don't know if the product is significant because there is an interaction between the risk factors or because the risk of outcome is significantly higher when both risk factors are present (compared to subjects who do not have both risk factors). In this example, if the investigators did not include the separate variables for male gender and ST elevations, and entered only the product term, the product term certainly would have been statistically significant and positive (since males with ST elevations are at higher risk of heart attack than the rest of the sample). But the importance of the product term is that it is statistically significant and negative when both male gender and ST elevations are in the model.

Although I have stressed the importance of initially including the variables that constitute the product term in the model, it would not be incorrect to have a model that had only the product term. If, for example, the two variables constituting the product term are not on their own statistically associated with the outcome in initial models, it would be acceptable to drop them from subsequent models.

An alternative method for incorporating product terms into your analysis is to create multiple dichotomous variables representing the

> Because a product term describes the relationship between two risk factors and an outcome, it can only be interpreted as an interaction if the two risk factors are in the model.

PERFORMING THE ANALYSIS

interaction. Look back at Table 8.2. There are four distinct codings of the variables gender and ST elevations. Rather than entering three variables representing gender, ST elevations, and the product of gender and ST elevations, you could create three dichotomous variables:

men with ST elevations (yes/no),
men without ST elevations (yes/no),
women with ST elevations (yes/no).

The reference group would be women without ST elevations. One advantage of this coding is that it will be easier for you to see and interpret the impact of the combinations of gender and ST elevations on outcome. A second advantage is that you can see the effect of the double exposed group (male and ST elevations) compared to persons with only one risk factor and persons with neither risk factor (the reference group). (When you use product terms you see the risk of the doubly exposed persons compared to persons with only one or no risk factors.)

A disadvantage of multiple dichotomous variable coding is that if you are looking at multiple interactions involving a particular variable (e.g., male gender) you will have to create more additional variables than you would if you were using product terms. For example, to describe the interaction between gender and congestive heart failure you would need three variables: men with congestive heart failure, men without congestive heart failure, and women with congestive heart failure. If you wanted instead to create an interaction term you would enter only two variables: congestive heart failure and the product of congestive heart failure and male gender. You would not have to add a variable for male gender because it is already in the model.

8.4 How do I enter time into my proportional hazards or other survival analysis?

For linear and logistic regression you need only enter your independent and dependent variables. For proportional hazards analysis and other types of survival analysis you must also enter a time for each subject. The time is the interval from a subject's participation in the study to the date the subject experienced an outcome, was lost to follow-up, was withdrawn, or completed the study.

The starting point ("zero time") will depend on the kind of study you are performing, as shown in Table 8.3. For a randomized controlled trial the starting time is the date of randomization. For a trial

TABLE 8.3
Starting time for survival study.

Type of study	Start time
Randomized controlled trial	Date of randomization
Nonrandomized trial	Enrollment into trial
Observational study	Varies:
	Date of first visit
	Date of first symptoms
	Date of diagnosis
	Date of start of treatment

that prospectively enrolls subjects but does not randomize them to a treatment, the starting point is usually the date of enrollment.

In observational studies, the choice of starting point is complicated. The goal is to choose a starting point that best represents the start of the process you are studying. For example, in evaluating the rate of death in patients with coronary artery disease, the starting point should be the onset of coronary artery disease. But how do you determine the date that coronary artery disease began? Is the starting point the date that the patient first developed chest pain? This sounds good, but remember some patients have coronary artery disease without ever having chest pain. Others have chest pain for years from some other cause before they develop coronary artery disease. Also, some patients will not remember their first episode of chest pain; they may report that they have had chest pain for "years."

What can you do to get a more precise starting time? You could use the date coronary angiography first demonstrated coronary artery stenosis. This starting date has the advantage of being the most objective (angiography is the gold standard for diagnosing coronary artery disease). But many patients never require angiography, and access to care and patients' willingness to undergo testing will affect whether and when they have angiography.

Often with observational studies, no one starting point truly represents the onset of the disease process for all participants. You have to choose the best one you have available. In a study of patients seen in a clinical setting this may be the date the patient first presented for medical care. In a prospective cohort study the starting point may be the first cohort visit. Although not ideal, date of first visit has been used in many studies. Notably, many natural history studies of HIV infection use the date of first visit because this was the first date that the participant was documented to be HIV-antibody positive. The actual disease process had begun months to years earlier when the person actually seroconverted to HIV. Although use of first visit did bias the results from these cohorts and has led to some inaccurate observations, these studies were nonetheless extremely helpful in understanding the nature of HIV disease.[51]

In conclusion, choose the starting point that best represents the start of the process you are studying and clearly state the choice in the methods section of your paper.

The endpoint for survival analysis is the date of the outcome of interest or the censor date (Section 7.3). For subjects lost to follow-up prior to outcome the censor date is the last date of known follow-up. For subjects who did not experience an outcome and were not lost to follow-up the censor date is the end date of the study (assuming intention-to-treat analysis for patients who are withdrawn).

In some studies there may be ambiguity about the appropriate censor date because the investigators have access to supplemental sources of data about study participants. Analysis of survival time following an AIDS diagnosis provides a good illustration of this principle. Let's say you want to determine whether persons who are lost to follow-up in your study have died. You know that death certificates are part of the public record and it is therefore possible to determine whether subjects who are lost to follow-up have died. However, you are also aware that there is usually a delay between when a subject dies and when you will learn about their death from a local, state, or national death registry. Conversely, matching with a death registry may enable you to learn about the deaths of some participants sooner than you otherwise would have. This can occur if you interview subjects only periodically (e.g., every six months to a year) but perform frequent reviews with a death registry (e.g., weekly to monthly). How should you deal with this supplementary information about survival?

---

[51] For a perspective on the biases of prevalent cohorts of HIV-infected persons see Alcabes, P., Pezzotti, P., Phillips, A.N., Rezza, G., Vlahov, D. "Long-term perspective on the prevalent-cohort biases in studies of human immunodeficiency virus progression." *Am. J. Epidemiol.* 1997;146:543–51.

In San Francisco, we follow all persons who are diagnosed with AIDS by reviewing their medical records every six months. We also review all of the death certificates in San Francisco weekly. Each year we perform a match with the National Death Index.[52] This index covers the deaths of all persons in the United States. Thus, when someone dies we almost certainly find out about it. We need to decide what is the appropriate date to use as the last date of follow-up for someone who is not known to have died. The algorithm we use to determine this date is somewhat complicated but illustrates the types of decisions you must make about the last date of follow-up.

For subjects not known to have died, we check the medical record for the date of the last medical visit or laboratory test. What about people whose records show no recent entries and yet are not listed as being dead? These people either died outside San Francisco (because if they died in San Francisco we would know it since we do weekly reviews of San Francisco's death certificates), moved, switched their site of care, or stopped receiving medical care altogether. What should our last date of follow-up be for these individuals?

For persons not known to have died, with no recent medical follow-up, we use for their censor date the date to which the National Death Index is current at the time we match our database with theirs. The National Death Index receives all state death certificates and updates their computer files for the deaths that occurred in a calendar year within twelve months of the end of the calendar year. For example, if we performed our match in June of 1999, the data would be complete for the calendar year of 1997. For those cases lost to follow-up, we would use December 31, 1997 as the censor date.

Of course, matches with the National Death Index are not perfect. The index is not 100% complete (nothing ever is). Also, it is possible that a case is listed in the National Death Index but we are unable to match with it because we have incorrect identifying information (e.g., the wrong date of birth). A more conservative strategy than using the date for which the National Death Index is current would be to use the last date listed in the medical record for those patients not known to have died. The problem with this strategy is that it underestimates survival because it counts those deaths that we know occurred after

---

[52] Applications for matching your data with the National Death Index can be obtained by writing or calling: National Death Index, Division of Vital Statistics, National Center for Health Statistics, 6525 Belcrest Road, Room 840, Hyattsville, MD 20782, 301-436-8951.

the last date of follow-up, but not the survival time beyond the date of follow-up. At the other extreme, we could censor everyone at the date of analysis. Supporting this strategy is the fact that most San Francisco AIDS patients die in San Francisco and we review the death certificates weekly. Therefore, in most cases we will know promptly if someone has died. However, using the date of analysis would overestimate survival because it would count all of the follow-up time but would miss some of the deaths. Our method is something of a compromise.

As you can see, the date of censor can be quite a complicated issue. Your choice will affect the survival time. van Benthem and colleagues illustrate this using a similar example to mine, that of AIDS incubation time (time from HIV seroconversion to AIDS diagnosis).[53] In their example, they show that AIDS incubation time varies based on whether you censor everyone at their last visit (because it does not use any supplementary information) or censor everyone at the date that they conduct the match with their local AIDS registry (overestimates survival because it assumes the local AIDS registry is complete). In their example, they advocate for an alternative method: Persons seen in the prior year, who are not in the AIDS registry, are assumed to be AIDS-free; persons not seen in the prior year and persons who developed AIDS more than a year after their last date of follow-up are assumed to be AIDS-free one year after their last date of follow-up.

Perhaps the most interesting thing about the analysis of van Benthem and colleagues is that they demonstrate that differences in AIDS incubation time reported by different studies may actually be due to differences in the censoring techniques. Thus, in handling supplementary information, I recommend you balance information about outcomes with information about outcome-free time and try to be consistent with how others in your field have dealt with this issue.

Once you have settled on the start date and end date for each subject, the difference between these dates represents the survival time for each subject in your analysis.

Table 8.4 illustrates calculations of time for different types of subjects. Subjects were enrolled between May 1, 1995 and August 1, 1995 and were followed until August 1, 1996 unless they dropped out or were withdrawn. The outcome of interest is heart attack.

> **✓ TIP**
>
> Choose a censor date that balances information about outcomes with information about outcome-free time.

[53] van Benthem, B.H.B., Veugelers, P.J., Schecter, M.T., Kaldor, J.M., Page-Shafer, K.A., van Griensven, G.J.P. "Modelling the AIDS incubation time: Evaluation of three right censoring strategies." *AIDS* 1997;11:834–5.

TABLE 8.4

Illustration of time calculations for individual subjects.

Subject	Start Date	Did heart attack occur?	Date of heart attack	Date of last follow-up	Time (days)
#1	May 1, 1995	Yes	May 1, 1996	August 1, 1996	365
#2	May 1, 1995	No	Not applicable	August 1, 1996	455
#3	August 1, 1995	No	Not applicable	August 1, 1996	365
#4	May 1, 1995	No	Not applicable	July 1, 1995	60

Subject #1 experienced a heart attack one year (365 days) after enrollment but continued to be followed after the outcome. This is common in clinical studies. You might follow someone beyond their main outcome of interest because you are assessing the development of side effects or a secondary outcome (e.g., death). However, note that to determine time to heart attack for this analysis, you subtract the start date from the date of outcome, not the date of last follow-up. Let's contrast this with subject #2. This subject did not have a heart attack. Therefore time is the difference between the start date and the date of last follow-up. Subject #3, like subject #2, did not experience a heart attack. But this subject enrolled in the study later than subjects #1 and #2. Therefore, even though the subject stayed till the end of the study, the subject would be censored at 365 days. Subject #4 dropped out of the study and is censored at 60 days.

The four subjects shown in Table 8.4 illustrate two important points about survival analysis.

- Survival analysis tracks length of time without reference to calendar time. If you changed the decade in which the study occurred by subtracting ten years from all the dates, you would get the same survival time. This is the reason that many analyses adjust for year of diagnosis or birth cohort (i.e., year or period of years of birth).
- There is no special designation for cases that are censored. All subjects that do not experience an outcome are censored. The only difference between subjects #2, #3, and #4, from the computer's point of view, is the amount of time they contribute to the analysis.

There is another method for incorporating time into a proportional hazards model: Use of age of subject rather than study time. Using age instead of study time makes sense in observational studies of healthy persons. This is because the hazard of an outcome such as death for a 55-year-old man observed for 15 years is likely to be more similar to the hazard for a 55-year-old man observed for 5 years, than that for a 40-year-old man observed for 15 years.

Korn and colleagues argue persuasively for the use of age instead of study time for observational studies of healthy persons drawn from national surveys.[54] However, their empirical analysis demonstrates that the more usual method of study time, with adjustment for subject's age, produces unbiased estimates even when age may be a more appropriate time scale.

Although the use of age in place of study time has its adherents, it is not commonly done, even for surveys of healthy persons. It would certainly not be appropriate in studies of persons with disease. In persons with an illness (e.g., cancer, heart disease) the amount of time that they have the disease is likely to be a more important predictor of their rate of outcome (e.g., death) than their age.

If you do choose to use age as your time scale, it is important to adjust for birth cohort. Otherwise, your model will not take into account treatment changes that have occurred during the lives of your participants.

8.5 What about subjects who experience their outcome on their start date?

It sometimes happens that subjects experience their outcome on their start date. If this occurs, the time for such subjects would be zero. Since, at time zero, by definition, none of the subjects have experienced an outcome, persons with time equal to zero must be excluded from the analysis. Is this fair? Can you do anything to prevent this?

To answer this question, you have to distinguish those cases where the outcome truly occured on the start date from those cases where the start date and the outcome are *recorded* as occurring on the same date, but the start date is really unknown. I will illustrate with a few examples.

---

[54] Korn, E.L., Graubard, B.I., Midthune, D. "Time-to-event analysis of longitudinal follow-up of a survey: Choice of the time scale." *Am. J. Epidemiol.* 1997;145:72–80.

Imagine you are studying hospital survival with a rapidly progressive disease, such as adult respiratory distress syndrome (ARDS). A certain number of patients will die on their day of admission to the hospital. In this case, if you computed survival in days, patients who died on their date of admission would appear to have a survival of zero days and would be excluded from the analysis. Clearly, this is not what you would want. The true survival time for these patients is in hours. Our use of a day as the unit of survival analysis is arbitrary. For this example, you should switch your unit of analysis to hours. This will work well for ARDS or other diseases that have a very rapid progression time. Day is the convention for most survival analyses because improvement and worsening of most clinical conditions occur in days not in hours.

Consider a more complex example: How to categorize patients who are diagnosed with AIDS and die on the same day. If you were to review data from the San Francisco Health Department's AIDS registry, you would discover that some of our cases have the same date for AIDS diagnosis and death. There are two reasons for this. In some cases, HIV-infected patients without an AIDS diagnosis are admitted to the hospital, diagnosed with an AIDS-defining illness for the first time, and die the same day they are admitted. In this case, as with the ARDS example, there is a real survival time, measured in hours. Unfortunately, our records do not contain the hour of AIDS diagnosis or death. In other cases, the patient's date of diagnosis is the same as their date of death because they are diagnosed by the medical examiner (coroner). In these cases, it is unclear what the true survival time is because you don't know if they had an AIDS illness for a short or a long time before death. How do we deal with these two types of cases, both of who have a survival time of zero?

For cases diagnosed on the day of admission, we consider their survival to be 0.5 days. The half day acknowledges that the death truly occurred after the diagnosis of AIDS, but after an interval of less than one day. (Some statistical software programs will automatically add 0.5 units to cases with a survival time of zero. However, you as the investigator should determine whether this is a reasonable assumption or not.) For those cases diagnosed by the medical examiner, we exclude the case because we do not know what the true interval is between diagnosis and death.

The AIDS registry of the New York City Health Department has an even more complicated problem. Unlike San Francisco, they only record the month and year of AIDS diagnosis. Thus a case who died in the same calendar month as their AIDS diagnosis would have a survival time of zero. They therefore have a large proportion of cases (11%) with survival time of zero.[55]

How do the investigators deal with New York City AIDS cases with survival time equal to zero? They exclude them from the analysis. This may be problematic. To the extent that such persons truly had short survival, their method will artificially lengthen survival by excluding these subjects. Because such cases represented a large group, the investigators assessed whether the survivors were different from other participants. In fact they were: They were more likely to be female, persons of color, and injection drug users. This illustrates another important point. You cannot always eliminate bias whether due to loss of cases or some other reasons. Nonetheless, you should always investigate it and describe it to your readers (as these authors did).

8.6 What about subjects who have a survival time shorter than physiologically possible?

It sometimes happens that a subject experiences their outcome so soon after their start date that the survival time is not physiologically possible. This is most likely to pose a dilemma with slowly progressive diseases, for which the physiology of the disease does not support a survival time of a day or a week. For example, what do you do with a subject enrolled in a study of cancer incidence who is diagnosed with lung cancer a week after enrollment? We know it takes years from the first malignant cell division to the time that the cancer is detectable. Do you exclude the subject who is diagnosed with cancer a week after enrollment? If you say yes, what about the subject diagnosed a month after, or a year after? The longer the time, the murkier the decision.

As with most things, prevention is the best defense. To avoid this problem, develop rigorous pre-enrollment criteria to ensure that subjects do not have the outcome at the time the study starts (at least as best as can be determined). Staying with the example of lung cancer, you may want subjects to have a respiratory symptom review and a pre-enrollment chest x-ray.

Unfortunately, certain diseases are difficult to rule out without subjecting participants to very invasive tests (which would increase

> ✓ **TIP**
>
> Develop rigorous pre-enrollment criteria to ensure that subjects do not have the outcome at the time the study starts.

---

[55] Blum, S., Singh, T.P., Gibbons, J., et al. "Trends in survival among persons with acquired immunodeficiency syndrome in New York City." *Am. J. Epidemiol.* 1994; 139:351–61.

the expense of your trial and decrease enrollment). For example, some HIV-infected patients have *pneumocystis carinii* pneumonia (PCP) with minimal or no symptoms and normal chest x-rays. If you wanted to be sure that subjects do not have PCP prior to enrolling them in a PCP prevention trial, you would have to perform bronchoscopy on all of them. However, it is not feasible or ethical to subject asymptomatic persons to an invasive test prior to enrollment in a trial to prevent the disease. Instead, most investigators performing studies on preventing PCP limit the pre-enrollment evaluation to a chest x-ray and symptom review. Invariably, a few patients are diagnosed with PCP just days after enrollment.

Besides being difficult to diagnose, PCP usually develops slowly, over a period of weeks. If a patient is diagnosed with PCP a week after starting a treatment protocol designed to prevent PCP, should the patient be considered a treatment failure (since the outcome of interest occurred while the patient was on the study) or should the subject be deleted from the analysis (since the subject almost certainly had PCP at the time of enrollment)? This is a judgment call. What most investigators do is to exclude those cases of PCP that occur within twenty-eight days of enrollment.[56] Cases that occur after twenty-eight days are considered treatment failures.

In considering this example you may wonder: Would it not be safer to include people who develop PCP after enrollment in the study no matter how soon after the start date? In support of this, remember that in a randomized controlled trial implausibly early outcomes should be evenly distributed in the different arms of the study. Therefore, including these early-outcome subjects will not bias your analysis, although it will result in your reporting higher treatment failure rates in the different arms of the study. But, in observational studies, improbably early outcomes would not necessarily be evenly distributed in the different arms of your study and could thus be a source of bias in your study.

My general advice in this area is develop pre-enrollment criteria that will lower the chance of implausibly early outcomes. Beyond this, decide ahead of time what you will do if a subject develops the outcome of interest a day after your study begins. If it will be important

> ✓ **T I P**
>
> Even if you have *a priori* criteria for exclusion it is best to have the decision to exclude a subject made by a review committee that is blind to the treatment assignment.

---

[56] Leung, G.S., Feigal, D.W., Montgomery, A.B., et al. "Aerosolized pentamadine for prophylaxis against *pneumocystis carinii* pneumonia." *N. Engl. J. Med.* 1990;323:769–75. Golden, J.A., Katz, M.H., Chernoff, D.N., Duncan, S.M., Conte, J.E. "A randomized comparison of once-monthly or twice-monthly high-dose aerosolized pentamadine prophylaxis." *Chest* 1993;104:743–50.

PERFORMING THE ANALYSIS

to you to exclude such early outcomes develop objective exclusion criteria for subjects prior to the start of a study. Even if you have a priori criteria for exclusion it is best to have a review committee that is blind to the treatment assignment make the decision to exclude a subject.

At times, it may be worth excluding early outcomes as a way of testing a hypothesis on the cause and effect relationship between your predictor and outcome. For example, in the study of cholesterol level and mortality discussed in Section 5.5, the investigators excluded cancers that occurred in the first four years of the study. They did this to test whether low cholesterol levels might be a consequence of cancer that was present but unsuspected at the time of entry into the cohort. When they excluded these cases, the relationship between low cholesterol level and cancer persisted, suggesting that the relationship between the low cholesterol level and mortality was not a consequence of unsuspected cancer at the time of enrollment.

8.7 What should I do about missing data on my independent variables?

Missing data is a problem in all types of analyses. However, the problems caused by missing data in bivariate analysis are magnified in multivariable analysis. Why? Because different subjects will likely have missing values on different variables. Imagine a study of 300 persons with 10 independent variables. Each variable has 10 missing subjects. In bivariate analysis, the sample size (N) will be 290 persons or 97% of your study population. But in multivariable analysis, there will likely be significantly more than 10 missing subjects because cases will be dropped from the analysis if they have a missing value on any of the independent variables. At one extreme, if each of the 10 variables is missing a different 10 subjects, you will lose 10 cases per variable, or 100 cases for ten variables. Your N will be 200 or only 66% of your study population. With this amount of missing data, your power to find a significant result is less. Furthermore, your results may not be generalizable to the study population if the missing cases are systematically different from those cases where the data are not missing.

Usually, subjects who have missing values on one variable are more likely to have missing values on other variables. Therefore, the number of cases that will need to be dropped will likely be less than 100. How much less depends on how many cases have missing values on more than one independent variable. The opposite extreme from my example would be if all ten variables had missing values for the

> The problems caused by missing data in bivariate analysis are magnified in multivariable analysis.

> **TABLE 8.5**
> Methods for dealing with missing data in multivariable analysis.
>
> ---
>
> 1. Delete cases with any missing data.
> 2. Create dichotomous variables to represent missing data.
> 3. Make additional effort to obtain data.
> 4. Decrease the number of independent variables in the analysis.
> 5. Estimate the value of the missing cases.

✓ **T I P**

To determine how many missing cases you will have in your multivariable analysis, create a variable whose value is "1" if data are missing on any independent variable.

✓ **T I P**

To assess bias due to cases with missing values, compare persons with missing data to persons without missing data on the important independent and dependent variables of your study.

same ten cases, in which case your multivariable analysis would have no more missing data than your bivariate analysis.

In preparation for deciding how you will deal with missing data in your analysis, it is often helpful to know ahead of time how many missing cases you will have in your multivariable analysis. To determine this, create a variable whose value is 1 if data are missing on any independent variables in your analysis and 0 if all the data are present. A simple frequency will then tell you how many cases will be missing in a multivariable analysis that includes all of these variables.

After you have determined how much missing data you have, what can you do? Table 8.5 shows five methods for dealing with missing data on independent variables in multivariable analysis. These are discussed in what follows.

Deleting cases with missing values on any independent variable is certainly straightforward and remains the most common method of dealing with missing data in clinical research. However, deleting cases with missing values may introduce bias into your analysis if the cases with missing data are different from cases without missing data (less compliant with filling out forms, less trusting of interviewers, cognitively impaired, etc.).

Although it may be impossible to eliminate bias due to excluded cases, it is possible to assess the likelihood of such bias. To do this, compare persons with and without missing data on the important independent and dependent variables of your study. If there are significant differences between persons with missing data and those without, you can report these differences, so as to better characterize the potential bias in your study. If there are no differences, you can feel better about excluding these cases, but recognize that there still may be bias due to unmeasured factors. Characterizing how missing cases differ from nonmissing cases is also useful information prior to estimating missing values (method #5).

You will note that assessing bias due to missing cases is similar to assessing bias introduced by subjects choosing not to participate in a study (response bias). Ironically, although the bias introduced by excluding cases with missing data is of equal importance as the bias introduced by nonparticipation, it is much less often reported in published reports. Of course, if you are missing only a few cases, it may not be necessary to evaluate the bias introduced by excluding them.

If you plan on deleting cases in your multivariable analysis that have missing values on any independent variable, you will have to decide how you want to deal with these cases in the univariate and bivariate analyses. You have two choices: You can exclude such cases right from the start of your analysis or you can wait until starting the multivariable analysis.

In published clinical research reports investigators tend to exclude such cases right from the start. The advantage of this method is that all analyses (univariate, bivariate, and multivariable) in the report then have the same sample size. The disadvantage is that much can be learned from univariate and bivariate analysis. It seems pointless to delete cases from a univariate or bivariate analysis just because they are missing on some other variable that will be part of the multivariable analysis. However, it does make it harder to follow the published analysis if the sample size changes for each analysis.

If the missing data are scattered over a large number of variables it is reasonable to delete cases with missing data on any independent variable. However, if one or two variables account for most of the missing data, it is not worth the loss of a large number of cases on the univariate and bivariate analysis to have the same sample size on all analyses. Remember, if you don't exclude the cases with missing values right from the start of the analysis, you should be careful to tell the reader the sample size for each analysis.

> **✓ TIP**
>
> If you don't exclude the cases with missing values right from the start of the analysis, be sure to tell the reader the sample size for each analysis.

A second strategy for handling missing data is to create multiple dichotomous variables (as you would with a nominal variable), with one variable signifying persons with missing data. This strategy was used for dealing with missing data in a study of determinants of kidney transplant failure.[57] The investigators coded the variable, amount of

---

[57] Chertow, G.M., Milford, E.L., Mackenzie, H.S., Brenner, B.M. "Antigen-independent determinants of cadaveric kidney transplant failure." *JAMA* 1996; 276:1732–6.

cold ischemia time, as six dichotomous variables: 9–16 hours (yes/no), 17–24 hours (yes/no), 25–36 hours (yes/no), 37–48 hours (yes/no), greater than 48 hours (yes/no), and missing value (yes/no). The reference group was 0–8 hours.

The advantage of using a dichotomous variable to indicate missing data is that it allows all subjects to be included in the multivariable analysis, without making a strong assumption about the missing subjects' values. It has the additional advantage that you get some sense of the bias introduced due to missing data. In the case of the kidney transplant study, those "yes" on the missing variable had the highest risk of graft failure. This would suggest that those with missing values actually had cold ischemia times greater than the other categories (since long cold ischemia time was associated with higher rates of graft failure). The authors also reported that the fit of models that included a dichotomous variable representing those cases with a missing value on cold ischemia time were not significantly different from the fit of models that excluded cases with missing data.

Since this book is primarily about data analysis, it may surprise you that I have listed "additional effort to obtain data" as the third strategy for dealing with missing data. Won't it be too late to go back to obtain additional data once you are already in the data analysis phase? Certainly, the data collection phase is the most appropriate and efficient time to obtain complete data. I mention this strategy here because the impact of missing data is often felt most acutely in the data analytic phase and sometimes researchers are subsequently able to obtain data that were previously missing. In the case of one study I was involved in, the missing data were in another city. When a thoughtful reviewer pointed out the weakness in our study caused by the missing data, we sent a research assistant on a trip to obtain the data. Some of you may complain that we should have sent a research assistant to collect the data from the other city right from the start. But, research, like any enterprise, is a series of trade-offs between costs (e.g., time, travel) and gains (e.g., more data). It was only after the variable proved to be so important to the analysis (and to the odds that the paper would be published!) that it seemed worth the effort and expense to get the data.

The fourth method for dealing with missing data, decreasing the number of independent variables in the analysis, works only if you have variables that can be eliminated without compromising your analysis. In Section 7.2, I discussed strategies for decreasing the number of independent variables in instances where your sample size is insufficient for the number of variables in your analysis. These strategies can also help with missing data. There are a few differences worth mentioning. Usually, some variables have more missing data than other variables in the study. Those variables with a large number of missing observations are the variables you should try to eliminate. If you have two related variables and one has a lot more missing data than the other, exclude the one with the greater number of missing observations. For example, education and income are highly correlated. If you have education level for everyone but income level for only 75% of the subjects (people are more sensitive about disclosing income than education level), it may be preferable to drop income and use only educational level in the analysis. Since income is not the same as educational level you will certainly lose information by doing this. Only you as the researcher can answer the question of whether you lose more by dropping the cases or by dropping the variable.

Variable selection techniques can also help you deal with missing data (Section 8.9). How? After the variables have been selected, rerun the model restricted to the selected variables. By decreasing the number of variables, you will likely decrease the number of cases that have to be excluded due to their having a missing value on at least one independent variable. To illustrate, say you have a sample size of 100 and ten independent variables, each of which has two cases with missing data; no one case has a missing value on more than one variable. Say you use backward elimination (a procedure that sequentially deletes variables from the model based on the association of the variables with outcome; Section 8.9). Because the model requires data on all variables to perform the backward elimination your model is based on a sample size of 80 ($100 - (10 \times 2)$). The model eliminates six variables that are not strongly associated with your outcome, leaving you with a model with four variables. You then rerun your model with only those four variables in it. The sample size will now be 92 ($100 - (4 \times 2)$) because cases that are missing on the six variables that are no longer in your analysis will not be excluded. Forward selection (a procedure that sequentially adds variables to the model based on the association of the variables with outcome; Section 8.9) can be used in a similar way. For example, if the forward selection chooses four variables from the original ten, run a fixed model using only these four variables.

For those of you who are even more compulsive, you can use backward elimination and rerun the model after each step, rather than waiting for the final solution. The advantage of this technique is that each step of your backward elimination will be based on a larger sample

> ✓ **TIP**
>
> Variable selection techniques can help with missing data. After the variables are chosen, rerun the model with the more restricted number of independent variables.

TABLE 8.6
Methods of estimating missing values.

For cross-sectional data:

Assign the sample mean.

Assign the mean by subgroup (conditional mean).

Model the value of the missing data by using the other covariates in the analysis (simple imputation).

Model the value of the missing data by using the other covariates in the analysis and include a random component (multiple imputation).

For longitudinal data with repeated measurements of the subjects:

Carry the last observation forward.

Model the missing observation based on serial values.

---

size, increasing the chance that the model is eliminating (and retaining) the "right" variables.

Rerunning your analysis by including only those variables selected in the original model should produce similar variable coefficients as your original model but narrower confidence intervals (because the sample size is larger). If there are significant differences between the models, it suggests that subjects with missing data are different from those without missing data.

The fifth method for dealing with missing data, estimating the value of missing cases, is the most satisfying but also the most dangerous method. It is more satisfying because you don't lose any cases; it is more dangerous because you may bias your results in ways that are difficult to predict. Several methods of estimating missing values for cross-sectional and longitudinal studies are shown in Table 8.6.

The simplest method of assigning a missing value for an independent variable is to assign the sample mean (or median) for that variable. (Choose the median if the distribution is skewed.) By assigning the mean/median you are saying that you believe the missing data are occurring randomly and therefore the mean/median provides the best estimate. The benefit of this procedure is that you get to keep the case with missing data in your analysis. However, this method is only sensible if the subjects for which you are assigning the mean/median have only one or two independent variables with missing values. If, for example, you have fifteen cases that have missing values on only one of ten independent variables, by assigning the mean/median for the missing variable you keep all fifteen cases in your analysis. They are useful cases because the information on the other nine independent variables is real. Viewed from the other extreme, if you have fifteen cases with missing values on all ten variables, it would serve no purpose to assign them the mean for each of the ten variables. Since all of the data on the independent variables are missing, they contribute no information to your multivariable analysis. Therefore prior to assigning values to missing data make sure that the cases have true values for at least half of the independent variables in your analysis.

When you assign missing values, you may want to assign mean/median values by subgroups rather than using the mean/median for the entire sample. This procedure is referred to as a conditional mean (conditional on the value of other variables). For example, if you have a number of cases with missing data on income, rather than assigning the mean/median for the whole sample, you may assign these cases the mean/median for other subjects of the same educational level and occupational status. Since income is correlated with educational attainment and occupational status, assigning the mean/median by subgroup will likely yield more accurate estimates of missing values.

✓ **T I P**

Conditional means will likely yield more accurate estimates of missing values than sample means.

A more sophisticated method of predicting the mean is to perform a multiple linear or logistic regression analysis using the other independent variables to predict the missing value. This method, usually referred to as imputation, may allow a more precise estimate of the missing value. However, as with all the above methods of estimating missing values, if you use the estimated values in your multivariable analysis you will underestimate the error associated with your coefficients. The reason is that once you have filled in the missing values based on your regression analysis, the computer does not know that the filled-in values have more "error" than those values that are actually observed. This results in confidence intervals surrounding the estimates that underestimate the actual variability of those estimates.

To overcome this problem, multiple imputation methods allow you to add in a random component.[58] With multiple imputation, you fit a multiple regression or logistic model for the variable with

✓ **T I P**

Multiple imputation methods allow you to estimate a missing value while adding in a random component.

---

[58] Heitjan, D.F. "What can be done about missing data? Approaches to imputation." *Am. J. Pub. Health* 1997;87:548–50.

missing values using subjects with complete data on this variable and its important correlates. The fitted model provides an estimate of the mean and variance of each missing value given the data on the correlates available for that subject. Next, for each missing value, you use a random number generator to simulate an observation from the estimated distribution, under the assumption that interval variables are normally distributed and that dichotomous variables have a binomial distribution. Then the primary analysis is carried out using this data set completed by the imputed missing values. This procedure is repeated at least ten times, and the results are combined using available formulas.[59] Repeating the procedure makes it possible to compute standard errors that take into account the extra uncertainty induced by the imputation, since each data set is completed with different imputed values for the missing data.

For longitudinal studies, where you have serial measurements of the independent variables for your subjects, you have additional options for estimating missing data. The simplest is to carry the prior (i.e., most recent) observation forward. The assumption here is that the best estimate of a missing observation is the observation immediately preceding it.

A more sophisticated method for serial measurements is to model the missing value based on prior, subsequent, or both prior and subsequent values. For example, in studies of HIV infection it is common to assess CD4 lymphocyte counts on sequential visits. Several investigators have faced the question of what to do with subjects who have one missing CD4 count. It would be a waste of data to delete a subject that had a CD4 count performed at time 0, time 6 months, time 18 months, and time 24 months, just because the participant was unavailable for monitoring at 12 months. Since CD4 lymphocyte counts had been shown to decrease in a linear fashion over time (prior to the development of highly effective antiretroviral therapy), one common technique was to estimate missing CD4 count values by drawing the best regression line for that case's CD4 counts over time. The estimated value at the missing point (in the case of this example, at 12 months) can then be used in further analyses.

Since each method of dealing with missing values has its advantages and disadvantages, some studies will use a combination of methods. For example, Halfon and colleagues conducted a study on access

---

[59] Rubin, D.B. *Multiple Imputation for Nonresponse in Surveys*. New York: Wiley, 1987.

to health services among Latino children.[60] Income was not reported for 13% of the sample. They estimated income by replacing missing values with the sample mean. In addition, they created a dichotomous variable representing the cases with missing data on income (in other words, the variable equals 1 if cases are missing and 0 if the cases are not missing). In this way, they were able to provide a value for income for their entire sample and adjust for the possibility that the cases with missing data were different from those without missing data.

One advantage of trying a variety of methods for dealing with missing data (e.g., eliminate cases, assign the mean, impute values) is that you can see if your choice of method makes a difference in the results. It is reassuring to researchers and to readers when different methods of dealing with missing data produce similar findings.

My general guidance on this complicated issue is:

1. Collect your data to minimize missing information.
2. Assess how much missing data you have on individual independent variables.
3. If you have one or two independent variables that have significantly more missing cases than your other variables, consider deleting the variables rather than the cases. No matter how important the variable is to your theory, if you have a lot of missing data on that variable, your information is likely biased.
4. After you have minimized missing data through #1 and #3 above, check to see how many cases have missing values on any of the independent variables you are planning to use in your multivariable model. If you have few cases with missing data, delete them right from the start. It is easier to follow a paper that has the same sample size for all analyses.
5. If you have a large number of cases with missing data, determine if cases with missing values differ from cases without missing values.
6. If missing cases do not differ from nonmissing cases, consider assigning means or conditional means. Before you do this, make sure that the cases have true values for at least half of the independent variables in your analysis. If you have cases that are missing data on most of your independent variables, delete them. If you have good biostatistical backup consider using a multiple imputation approach.

[60] Halfon, N., Wood, D.L., Valdez, B., Pereyra, M., Duan, N. "Medicaid enrollment and health services access by Latino children in inner-city Los Angeles." *JAMA* 1997;277:636–41.

7. If missing cases differ from nonmissing cases, you are in a tough spot. Go forward as in #6, but be clear in your own mind, and to your readers, that assigning values based on the other cases is problematic since you know that the cases with missing values are not the same as nonmissing cases. Of course, excluding them is problematic for the same reason.
8. If possible, try more than one method for dealing with missing data.
9. Read more about the theory and practice of dealing with missing data.[61]

8.8 What should I do about missing data on my outcome variable?

Of those strategies listed in Table 8.6 for dealing with missing data on independent variables, only deleting cases and making additional effort to get the data will work reliably for a missing outcome variable. You can't eliminate your outcome variable (that is, what you are studying). You also cannot estimate your outcome variable prior to the multivariable analysis. The whole purpose of multivariable analysis is to estimate the outcome variable based on the independent variables. For longitudinal studies, persons who are lost to follow-up can contribute to the analysis by censoring observations (Section 7.3). However, it is best not to think of censored observations as missing outcome data. For a censored observation you know what the outcome is at a particular time. You just don't know the outcome beyond that time.

Although you cannot estimate your outcome variable prior to your multivariable analysis, you can use a multiple imputation technique to estimate it after your multivariable analysis. How? Remember that multivariable models estimate outcome based on the relationship of the independent variables to the outcome. Once you have estimated outcome based on cases where you have information on independent variables and outcome, you can estimate the outcome of cases where you only have information on the independent variables. What good

[61] Marascuilo, L.A., Levin, J.R. *Multivariate Statistics in the Social Sciences: A Researcher's Guide.* Monterey, CA: Brooks/Cole Publishing Co., 1983, pp. 64–6. Delucchi, K.L. "Methods for the analysis of binary outcome results in the presence of missing data." *J. Consult Clin. Psych.* 1994;62:569–75. Little, R.J.A., Rubin, D.B. *Statistical Analysis with Missing Data.* New York: Wiley, 1990. Greenland, S., Finkle, W.D. "A critical look at methods for handling missing covariates in epidemiologic regression analyses." *Am. J. Epidemiol.* 1995;142:1255–64.

does this do? By estimating the outcome variable for cases with missing outcomes and including a component that takes into account the variability of this estimate, you can repeat your multivariable analysis with the additional cases and see if your results differ. If they do not, it strengthens the validity of your analysis.

This procedure was used in an evaluation of an HIV prevention intervention tailored for young gay men.[62] The researchers assessed the sexual risk activities pre- and post-intervention. They found significant decreases in HIV risk activities between the pre- and post-assessment for the intervention group compared to the non-intervention group. However, of 191 young men who received the pre-intervention assessment, only 103 (54%) were available for the post-intervention assessment. This substantial loss of the sample raises questions about the validity of the observed differences.

Even more problematic for the researchers, there were significant differences between those subjects lost to follow-up and those not lost to follow-up. Could these differences, rather than the intervention, explain why there were decreases in sexual risk activities following the intervention? There is no way to definitively answer this question since the subjects were lost and we do not know their ultimate outcome. But we do know something about their pre-intervention behavior.

What the researchers did is to estimate outcome for those subjects who had both pre-intervention and post-intervention interviews using logistic regression analysis. They then used these models to estimate outcome for those cases without a post-intervention assessment. Next, using a multiple imputation procedure, they generated 100 data sets in which the missing outcomes were randomly imputed from the distribution of the missing value according to the logistic model and the observed baseline covariates for the subject. The treatment effect was estimated by the average of the effect estimates for each of the 100 data sets. The standard errors were corrected for the multiple imputation by a factor depending on the variance of the 100 effect estimates. The results of this repeated analysis were similar to those of the analysis in which these cases were excluded. While this strengthened the conclusion of the paper, it certainly does not exclude bias as the explanation of their findings.

---

[62] Kegeles, S.M., Hays, R.B., Coates, T.J. "The Mpowerment project: A community-level HIV prevention intervention for young gay men." *Am. J. Public Health* 1996;86:1129–36.

8.9 What are variable selection techniques? Which variable selection technique should I use?

Variable selection techniques are algorithms that determine which independent variables will be included in a multivariable model. They also can determine the order in which the variables enter the model. The parameters of the algorithms are determined by the investigator.

I have already referred to variable selection techniques as strategies for decreasing the number of independent variables in your analysis. This may be necessary because of insufficient sample size for the number of independent variables in your model (Section 7.2) or because of missing data (Section 8.7). Besides these two, the other major reason for using selection procedures is that you want to determine the minimum number of independent variables necessary to accurately estimate outcome. This is particularly important in the development of diagnostic models (Section 2.1.D) because the fewer the variables the more likely clinicians are to remember and use them.

In Section 2.1.D, I detailed a decision rule for determining which patients presenting with chest pain to an emergency room were likely having acute ischemia. The investigators used forward stepwise regression to create the prediction rule. Using forward selection they evaluated a total of fifty-nine clinical characteristics; the selection algorithm chose the seven variables that best accounted for ischemia. If instead the investigators developed a model using all fifty-nine characteristics, it would undoubtedly have had better diagnostic capability than the seven-variable model. But what clinician would use a fifty-nine variable model in a clinical setting? Patients would require hospital admission just so that their physician would have enough time to record the values of the fifty-nine clinical characteristics and compute each patient's probability of ischemia!

Most statistical software packages offer a variety of variable selection techniques (Table 8.7). What all selection methods have in common is that they use statistical criteria to decide which variables should enter the model and the order of the variables entering the model.

Using forward selection, the model will select the variable most strongly related to the outcome and enter it first into the model. In fact, you can predict which variable will enter first in a forward selection model by looking at your bivariate analysis. The variable with the strongest association with your outcome in the bivariate analysis will enter first. You will not be able to predict the second variable that will enter simply by looking at the bivariate analysis because the model

TABLE 8.7

Methods of variable selection.

Type of selection technique	Method	Advantages and disadvantages
Forward	Enters variables into the model sequentially. The order is determined by the variable's association with outcome (variables with strongest association enter first) after adjustment for any variables already in the model.	Best suited for dealing with studies where the sample size is small. Does not deal well with suppresser effects.
Backward	Deletes variables from the model sequentially. The order is determined by the variable's association with outcome (variables with weakest association leave first) after adjustment for any variables already in the model.	Better for assessing suppresser effects than forward selection.
Best subset	Determines the subset of variables that maximizes a specified parameter.	Computationally difficult.
None (All variables)	Enters all variables at the same time.	Including all variables may be problematic if there are many independent variables, a small sample size, or a lot of missing data.

will choose the variable that best improves the fit of the model after adjusting for the first variable. This may not be the second strongest predictor in bivariate analysis. It depends how closely these two independent variables are related to each other. If they are very closely related, it is possible that once you know the value of the first variable, the value of the second variable does not substantially improve the fit of your model. Instead a variable that is less strongly associated with outcome in the bivariate analysis, but unrelated to the first variable that entered, may be the second strongest variable in improving the fit of your model.

Forward selection will continue to evaluate each variable for how it improves the fit of your model. When none of the remaining variables significantly improve the fit, it will stop entering variables. You as the researcher decide what statistical cutoff to use for determining that the addition of another variable does not significantly improve the fit of the model. With lower cutoffs fewer variables will be included, but you will be more likely to miss important confounders. With higher cutoffs you will be less likely to miss important confounders but you will have a model with more variables in it.

Forward models can be modified to allow you to delete variables that were significant on entry into the model but are not statistically significant after other variables have entered. To do this, you will need to specify a statistical cutoff for removal of a variable that was already entered. You may want to set a less stringent (higher P value) cutoff to remove a variable once entered, or use the same cutoff for both. Forward selection models with deletion of entered variables that are no longer significant will produce a model with potentially fewer variables than simple forward selection.

Backward selection is similar to forward selection – except it proceeds backwards! At step one all variables enter into the model. If you have ten independent variables, all ten will enter in this step, no matter how unrelated they are to outcome. The algorithm then assesses which of the ten variables in the model is least important in accounting for the outcome, and deletes it, so that there are now nine variables in the model. The model then assesses which of the nine is least important in accounting for the outcome. It deletes this variable and then repeats the process until all the remaining variables are significantly associated with the outcome. At this point no further variables are deleted. As with forward selection, the researcher determines what statistical cutoff will be used for retaining (or not deleting) a variable.

You may, at first, think that forward or backward selection would arrive in the same place just by different routes, like two cars converging on a city from opposite directions. While it is a sign of a robust model when forward and backward selection give you the same answer, this does not always occur. The reason that forward and backward selection do not necessarily produce the same answer is that the importance of a particular variable often depends on what other variables are in the model at the time of selection. A variable may be statistically important when a variable (or a group of variables) is in the model and yet not significant when that variable (or group of variables) is not in the model. This is referred to as a suppresser effect (Section 1.3).

✓ **T I P**

Backward selection is more likely to demonstrate a suppresser effect than forward selection.

PERFORMING THE ANALYSIS

In forward selection, it is less likely that the variable needed to demonstrate the suppresser effect will be in the model. For this reason, backward selection is more likely to detect a variable that is significant only when the suppresser variable is in the model.

Forward selection is preferable over backward selection when your sample size is small for the number of independent variables in your analysis or when you have concerns about multicollinearity. This is because in backward selection all the variables are in the model initially. If you have doubts about the reliability of a model with all the variables in it, then there is reason to worry about having this model be the starting point for decisions on which variables to delete.

In best subset regression, the computer chooses the best combination of variables from all possible models. In the case of an analysis with only five variables, there are thirty-one possible combinations of variables (including models that have one, two, three, four, and five variables). The number of possible combinations increases exponentially as you increase the number of possible variables. "Best" is determined by a measure of the ability of the model to account for the outcome. For example, in multiple linear regression, you could have the computer choose the combination of variables that produces the highest adjusted R^2 (Section 9.2.B).

In some ways, best subset regression is hard to argue with. It is, after all, the best statistical answer to the question. However, because of the computational time involved, this technique cannot always be done. For logistic regression and proportional hazards analysis, best subset regression is usually modified to include the best possible combination of two variables, then of three variables, then of four variables, up to the maximum number of variables in your model (some programs will limit the maximum number of variables to ten). This is a simplification in that the computer is not comparing models of different size to one another (e.g., comparing those that have five variables to those that have four variables). Also, just because it is the best statistical answer does not mean it truly reflects the physiology of what you are studying. Confounders may be included in the model while the main effects are missing. Conversely, confounders that may change the coefficients of certain variables in important ways may be omitted.

Although I have described these selection algorithms as distinct, there are many hybrids. A popular hybrid is to enter certain variables in the model at the start of the analysis and not allow them to be deleted even if they are not significantly related to the outcome. The computer then enters the remaining independent variables in a forward

> ✓ **TIP**
>
> Forward selection is preferable to backward selection when your sample size is small for the number of independent variables in your analysis or when you have concerns about multicollinearity.

or backward manner. This strategy works well when there are certain variables that you absolutely want in your analysis for theoretical or practical reasons. For example, if every prior analysis of your outcome shows that age is an important confounder, it makes sense to add age right at the start, and not allow it to leave the model.

One of the criticisms of forward and backward models is that the criteria for inclusion or exclusion of a variable are based on that particular variable's statistical relationship with the outcome after adjustment for the other variables in the model. Instead, you might want to base decisions on whether to include a variable based on how its presence changes the other coefficients in the model. For example, you could enter variables one at a time into a model, and observe the difference that the variable makes to the other coefficients in the model. If inclusion of a variable has a major impact on other variables in your model (e.g., changes a variable coefficient by 10% or more) you would want to include it, even if it were not statistically associated with outcome. I alluded to this strategy in the discussion of how to limit the number of predictor variables in your model when you have a small sample (Section 7.2).

Forward and backward selection techniques can be modified to minimize the effect of missing data in your analysis. With forward or backward selection, after you have derived your model, you can rerun it with only the variables that entered (or were not deleted). By rerunning the model with a smaller number of variables, missing data on the excluded variables will no longer result in missing cases in the multivariable model. With backward selection, you can rerun the model with each deletion of a variable, so that each iteration of the model has a larger sample size (Section 8.7).

8.10 If I use a forward or backward selection technique, what level of statistical significance should I set for inclusion/exclusion of a variable?

Most researchers use a P value of $<.05$ or, for smaller sample sizes, a P value of $<.10$ or $<.15$. Of course, any cutoff is arbitrary. Just because a variable does not meet the P value criterion does not mean that it is unimportant. The algorithm does not evaluate whether entry of the variable changes the coefficients of the other variables in the model. While it is unlikely that a variable that has no association with outcome will make a significant impact on the other coefficients, it is possible that a variable that is marginally associated with the outcome will change the coefficients of the other independent variables in important ways. This is one reason many researchers favor higher (less restrictive) cutoffs than $P < .05$.

8.11 Do I have to use a variable selection technique at all?

Absolutely not. In fact, most researchers would agree that it is best not to use them. The decision of what variables to be included in a model is ideally made by the investigator, based on theoretical and empirical findings. With all of the variable selection models you run the risk of the model eliminating (or not selecting) a variable that is on the causal pathway to your outcome, in favor of a variable that is a confounder. Thus, I recommend that you do not use selection models unless you are trying to find the most parsimonious solution to your question or minimize the impact of missing data or have an insufficient sample size.

> Without selection criteria, all variables that you specify will be entered simultaneously. You will not have to worry about the possibility of missing suppresser effects or important changes in coefficients due to exclusion of a modest confounder. Another advantage of all variable models is that when you submit your paper for publication, you will not have to explain why certain variables are not included in your model. While one can certainly defend exclusion of a variable in selection models because it was not statistically related to the outcome, the reviewer may cite the possibility that the missing variable is a modest confounder or a suppresser variable. With an all variable model you can demonstrate that the variable of interest is included and does or does not affect the outcome and the relationship of the other independent variables to the outcome.

> ✓ **TIP**
> Don't use variable selection techniques unless: a) You are trying to find the most parsimonious solution to your question; b) you are trying to minimize the impact of missing data; or c) you have an insufficient sample size.

8.12 What value should I specify for tolerance in my logistic regression or proportional hazards model?

Tolerance is a measure of multicollinearity (Section 6.2). Very small values of tolerance indicate multicollinearity. If you have highly related variables in your analysis, the computer may be unable to solve the equation without deleting one or more of the problematic variables from the model. The default criteria set by your software package should work fine. In practice, this feature mainly works to delete completely redundant variables, such as when you create multiple dichotomous variables and include in the model a variable for the reference category (Sections 4.2 and 6.2).

> ⯈ **DEFINITION**
> *Tolerance* is a measure of multicollinearity.

8.13 How many iterations (attempts to solve) should I specify for my logistic regression or proportional hazards model?

The answer to this question is similar to the answer attributed to Abraham Lincoln when asked how long a man's legs should be: Long enough to reach the floor. You should set the number of iterations high enough to solve your equation (referred to as convergence of your model). A typical default value used by software packages is twenty-five attempts. It may take more attempts than that, especially if you have a small number of cases or skewed distributions for your independent or dependent variables (e.g., only three people are yes on a variable). Although the default will generally work, if it does not, increase the iterations until the model converges (solves the equation). However, note that when a higher number of iterations is required to get the model to converge there may be a problem with the model (Section 8.15).

8.14 What value should I specify for the convergence criteria for my logistic regression or proportional hazards model?

In multiple linear regression the parameter estimates can be found by solving an explicit system of equations. However, with logistic regression and proportional hazards models no such explicit solution exists. Instead, the maximum likelihood parameter estimates are found through a search algorithm. Starting from an initial rough solution, the algorithm modifies the estimates and recomputes the likelihood. The algorithm is determined to have converged on the maximum likelihood parameter estimates when the modifications increase the likelihood by less than the preset convergence criterion, or when the largest modification to any single parameter estimate falls below an analogous criterion. The defaults set by your software package should work fine.

8.15 My model won't converge. What should I do?

You may sometimes get a message that your logistic or proportional hazard models can't converge. What this means is that the computer cannot solve the equation. There are several reasons this can happen. In the simplest cases, you have made an error in your coding. If you have coded an outcome variable, such that everyone has the same outcome (this can happen if you are not careful with your if/then

PERFORMING THE ANALYSIS

statements), the computer cannot solve the equation. It cannot compute the odds of outcome versus no outcome if everyone has the outcome.

Recognizing this, you can probably imagine another reason that a model will not converge: You have too few outcomes for the number of independent variables in your model (Section 7.1). Your independent variables (e.g., smoking status, gender, age) may be defining subgroups for which there are no outcomes. For example it may be that among nonsmoking women under the age of forty-five years no heart attacks have occurred. Because this group has no members, the computer cannot determine the parameters for the variables of smoking status, gender, and age.

What can you do if your model won't converge and your outcome variable is correctly coded? You should check to see if your independent variables define any subgroups with no outcomes. If this is not the case, you can increase the number of attempts (iterations) the program makes to solve the equation. If increasing the iterations does not work, try decreasing the number of independent variables in your model so that there are no subgroups with very few outcomes. Removing independent variables that have very skewed distributions, especially less than 5% of subjects in a particular category, usually helps the most.

> ✓ **T I P**
>
> Models will not converge if you have defined a subgroup in which no (or very few) outcomes have occurred.

> ✓ **T I P**
>
> If your model does not converge even after increasing the number of iterations, try decreasing the number of independent variables in your model.

9

Interpreting the Analysis

9.1 What information will the printout from my analysis provide?

All three multivariable techniques will provide two kinds of information: information about the relationship of all independent variables taken together to the outcome and information about the relationship of each of the independent variables to your outcome variable (with adjustment for all other independent variables in your analysis). Let's review these in turn.

9.2 How do I assess how well my model accounts for my outcome?

As you can see in Table 9.1, there are a variety of methods of assessing how well your model accounts for your outcome.

9.2.A How do I know if my model (all my independent variables together) account for outcome better than I would expect by chance?

All three types of analyses provide a test of whether the independent variables, taken together, are more strongly associated with outcome than would be expected by chance. As is the case with all inferential statistics, you seek to disprove the null hypothesis. The null hypothesis in this case is that there is no relationship between the independent variables and the outcome. A significant relationship between the independent variables and the outcome means that you can reject the null hypothesis.

In multiple linear regression, the F test compares the success of the independent variables in accounting for the outcome compared

TABLE 9.1

Methods for measuring how well a model accounts for the outcome.

	Multiple linear regression	Multiple logistic regression	Proportional hazards analysis
Model accounts for outcome better than chance (Section 9.2.A)	F test	Likelihood ratio test	Likelihood ratio test
Quantitative/ qualitative assessment of how well model accounts for outcome (Section 9.2.B)	R^2	R^2 (rarely used), Comparison of estimated to observed value, Hosmer–Lemeshow test	Comparison of estimated to observed value
Prediction of outcome (Section 9.2.C)	Not applicable	Sensitivity, Specificity, Accuracy, c index	Not applicable

to the success in accounting for the outcome based on assuming that everyone in the study had the mean value for the outcome.[63] If knowing the values of the independent variables improves the fit more than would be expected by chance, then the value of F will be large. A large F value for a given sample size and a given number of variables in the model (which determines the degrees of freedom) will result in a small P value. This indicates that the null hypothesis of no association between the independent variables and the outcome can be rejected.

> If knowing the values of the independent variables improves the fit more than would be expected by chance, the null hypothesis can be rejected.

For multiple logistic regression and proportional hazards analysis, the test for assessing the significance of the overall model is the likelihood ratio test (often referred to as model chi-square). It is analogous to the F test. It has a chi-squared distribution.

---

[63] To see how F is calculated, see Glantz, S.A. *Primer of Biostatistics* (4th ed.). New York: McGraw-Hill, 1997, pp. 37–52.

For logistic regression the likelihood ratio test answers the question of whether the independent variables account for the outcome better than assuming the mean outcome for your subjects. Since logistic regression has a dichotomous outcome, the mean is simply the proportion of persons who experience an outcome. If knowing the values of the independent variables improves the fit of the model more than you would expect by chance, then the value of the chi-square will be large.

The likelihood ratio test answers a somewhat different question with proportional hazards analysis. With proportional hazards analysis, if the time to outcome of subjects with certain values on their independent variables are different from the baseline rate (more than you would expect by chance), then the chi-square will be large.

For both logistic regression and proportional hazards analysis, when the chi-square of the likelihood ratio test is large, for a given number of parameters in the model (degrees of freedom), the P value will be small. As with a large F test value, you will reject the null hypothesis and conclude that the independent variables are related to the outcome. The P value associated with the chi-square assumes a "large" sample size; sample sizes greater than 80–100 give a good approximation.[64]

Some limitations of the F and the likelihood ratio test will be apparent to you. They do not tell you which or how many variables in your model are significant. You can have a model with five variables in it, four of which are unassociated with the outcome, and still have a significant overall test. Methods for determining the importance of the individual variables are dealt with in Section 9.3.

Another limitation is that knowing that the variables as a group are more closely associated with outcome than you would expect by chance does not tell you quantitatively how well your independent variables account for outcome. Given these limitations, what are these tests useful for? If you get a global F or likelihood ratio test that is not significant you should worry that your model is a poor representation of your data. If individual variables are significantly related to outcome, and the overall model is not statistically significant, it suggests that there are many variables included in the model that are unrelated

> For both logistic regression and proportional hazards analysis, when the chi-square of the likelihood ratio test is large, the P value will be small and the null hypothesis can be rejected.

✓ **T I P**

If individual variables are significantly related to outcome but your overall model is not statistically significant, delete those variables that are not associated with outcome.

---

[64] For a more detailed explanation of the likelihood ratio test, see: Hosmer, D.W., Lemeshow S. *Applied Logistic Regression*. New York: Wiley, 1989, pp. 8–18; Menard, S. *Applied Logistic Regression Analysis*. Thousand Oaks, CA: Sage Publications, 1995, pp. 19–21.

to outcome. With each added variable, the degrees of freedom increase, and it takes a larger chi-square value to achieve a statistically significant result. Consider deleting variables from your model that are not associated with outcome.

9.2.B How do I assess how well my model accounts for my outcome?

A quantitative measure of how well the independent variables explain the outcome in multiple linear regression is R^2. R^2, also called the coefficient of variation, indicates how much better you can account for the outcome by knowing the values of the independent variables than by assuming that everyone had the mean value on the outcome variable.

The value of R^2 ranges from 0 (indicating that the independent variables do not explain the outcome any better than assuming everyone has the sample mean) to 1 (the independent variables completely account for the outcome). When R^2 is multiplied by 100 it can be thought of as the percentage of the variance in the dependent variable explained by the independent variables.

While R^2 is generally more informative than F, it has the limitation that its value will increase as you include additional independent variables, even if these variables add only a little bit of information. For example, a model with ten independent variables will have a higher R^2 than a model with five of these variables, even if the additional five variables add little to the model. To account for this, the statistic adjusted R^2 charges you a price for each variable in your model. As you add variables, adjusted R^2 can increase (the gain in having the variable is greater than the charge), decrease (the charge is greater than the gain), or stay the same (the gain and the charge are equal).

Although there is an R^2 measure for logistic regression, it does not perform as well for this type of analysis and is rarely reported in the literature. However, there are other methods for assessing how well the model accounts for the outcome.

A useful qualitative method for assessing a logistic regression model is to compare the estimated probability of outcome (according to the model) to the observed probability of outcome (the original data). To do this remember that the estimated probability is based on the pattern of independent variables for each subject. If your model has three variables, gender (male/female), age (in terciles), and hypertension (yes/no), then the number of distinct patterns of these three variables is $2 \times 3 \times 2 = 8$. In other words, whether you have ten subjects or

▶ DEFINITION

R^2 is a quantitative measure of how well the independent variables account for the outcome.

✓ TIP

When R^2 is multiplied by 100 it can be thought of as the percentage of the variance in the dependent variable explained by the independent variables.

Adjusted R^2 charges you a price for each variable in your model.

ten million there are only eight distinct patterns. For each of these patterns, there is an observed rate of outcome (the proportion of persons who experienced the outcome based on the data) and an estimated rate of outcome (based on the model).

If you have a large number of distinct covariate patterns, you can still use this technique by grouping patients with similar estimated likelihood of outcomes. Thus, for example, you may divide your sample into ten groups of estimated likelihood of outcome: 0–0.10, 0.11–0.20, etc. One problem with dividing estimated likelihood of outcome into equal divisions of likelihood is that you may still get small groups, if, for example, few persons have very high or very low estimated probabilities of outcome. Another alternative is to divide the probabilities such that there are approximately equal numbers of outcomes in each group.

The latter was done by Gordon and colleagues in a study of racial variation in predicted and observed in-hospital death rates.[65] The investigators used logistic regression to develop an estimated probability of in-hospital death. In their model, they included age, sex, race, type of health insurance, emergency department admission, and a mortality measure based on data from the first forty-eight hours of hospitalization. They divided the estimated risk of death into ten strata so that there would be equal numbers of outcomes in each group (653–654 deaths). Note that since the strata are based on the number of outcomes rather than the estimated risk of death, the different strata have varying widths of estimated risks of death (stratum 1 ranges from only 0.00 to 0.03 whereas stratum 10 ranges from .81 to 1.00). You can see that the estimated risk of death was similar to the observed probability of death in the ten strata (Table 9.2).

Although the data can be shown in tabular form, as was done by the authors in their article, the fit of the model can be seen a little better in Figure 9.1. I have created the figure from the data by plotting the midpoint of the estimated probability of death on the x axis against the observed probability of death along the y axis. You can see that the points (connected by a solid line) are all close to the dotted diagonal line, which represents perfect calibration.

If the points fall close to the diagonal, as in Figure 9.1, your model is an excellent estimate of outcome. If the points are scattered far from the line, it indicates that the model is not very accurate at estimating

[65] Gordon, H.S., Harper, D.L., Rosenthal, G.E. "Racial variation in predicted and observed in-hospital death." *JAMA* 1996;276:1639–44.

TABLE 9.2

Comparison of estimated to observed risk of death among hospitalized patients.

Stratum	Estimated risk of death	Observed risk of death
1	0.00–0.03	.01
2	0.03–0.06	.05
3	0.06–0.10	.09
4	0.10–0.17	.14
5	0.17–0.24	.24
6	0.24–0.34	.32
7	0.34–0.47	.38
8	0.47–0.63	.52
9	0.63–0.81	.66
10	0.81–1.00	.87

Adapted with permission from Gordon, H.S., et al. "Racial variation in predicted and observed in-hospital death." *JAMA* 1996;276:1639–44. Copyright 1996, American Medical Association.

observed outcomes. An advantage of this approach is that it also allows you to see if your model performs better at certain probabilities of disease.

For proportional hazards analysis, it is possible to compare estimated and observed time to outcome. This can be done using Kaplan–Meier survival curves for each important subgroup of patients defined by your model. For example, Colford and colleagues found in their proportional hazards analysis that two variables, CD4 count and hematocrit (both split at the median), had the strongest association with survival among HIV-infected patients with cryptosporidiosis.[66] To assess how well their model estimated survival, they stratified their

---

[66] Colford, J.M., Tager, I.B., Hirozawa, A.M., et al. "Cryptosporidiosis among patients infected with human immunodeficiency virus: Factors related to symptomatic infection and survival." *Am. J. Epidemiol.* 1996;144:807–16.

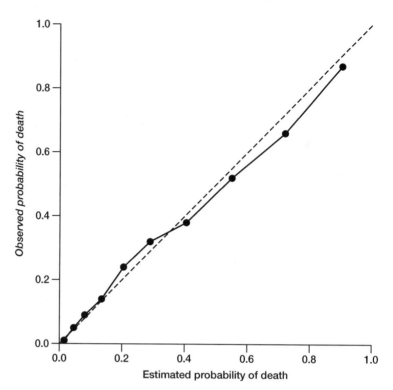

Figure 9.1. Estimated (x axis) versus observed values (y axis) for risk of death among hospitalized patients. Data from Gordon, H.S., Harper, D.L., Rosenthal, G.E. "Racial variation in predicted and observed in-hospital death." *JAMA* 1996;276:1639–44.

patients into four groups based on CD4 count and hematocrit. As shown in Table 9.3, they found that the estimated and observed median survival times were similar.

Because the underlying survival function is not automatically estimated in proportional hazards analysis, you need to use adjunct estimators to calculate estimated median survival. Also, this procedure will not work if there are few subjects who experienced the outcome. (To calculate an estimated median survival, half of the sample for each covariate pattern must experience the outcome.)

Comparing the estimated to observed probability, whether in tabular form (Table 9.2) or graphed (Figure 9.1), is a qualitative assessment of how well the model accounts for the outcome. There is a statistic that has been developed for logistic regression to assess how similar the estimated probability of outcome is to the observed probability of outcome. This statistic is called the Hosmer–Lemeshow goodness-

TABLE 9.3
Survival among subgroups of HIV-infected patients with Cryptosporidium.

Subgroup	Relative hazard	95% confidence interval	Median survival (days) Estimated	Median survival (days) Observed
CD4 count ≤53 cells/ml and hematocrit ≤37%	15.9	6.0–42.2	213	204
CD4 count ≤53 cells/ml and hematocrit >37%	8.1	2.8–23.6	465	341
CD4 count >53 cells/ml and hematocrit ≤37%	3.1	1.1–8.8	688	878
CD4 count >53 cells/ml and hematocrit >37%	1.0 (ref.)		1,119	1,119

Adapted with permission from Colford, J.M., et al. "Cryptosporidiosis among patients infected with human immunodeficiency virus." *Am. J. Epidemiol.* 1996;144:807–16.

of-fit test. The statistic compares the estimated to observed likelihood of outcome for groups of subjects. The groups are created by dividing the sample into approximately ten groups based on the range of estimated probability of outcome (the first group contains the 10% of subjects with the lowest estimated likelihood of outcome, the second group contains the 10% of subjects with the next lowest estimated likelihood of outcome, etc.). In a well-fitting model, the estimated likelihood will be close to the observed likelihood of outcome. This will result in a small chi-square and a nonsignificant *P* value.

9.2.C   How can I assess how well my model predicts the outcome of study subjects?

Because the outcomes in logistic regression are dichotomous, one can ask how well the model predicts the outcome of study subjects. To do this you must dichotomize the estimated outcome. In other words, you must choose a cutoff of what estimated probability of outcome you will consider to be a prediction of outcome. Once you do this, you can compute the sensitivity (proportion of persons who are predicted to have the outcome who really have it), specificity (proportion of persons who do not have the outcome who are predicted not to have it), and the proportion of correctly identified persons.

Choosing the cutoff for probability of outcome is not always easy. Each cutoff has a different sensitivity, specificity, and proportion of correctly identified persons. One simple cutoff is to assume that anyone with probability of outcome greater than 50% is predicted to have the outcome. However, the choice of 0.5 as the cutoff for measuring the predictive ability of your model may not be best. This is especially true for clinical diseases (e.g., ischemic heart disease) where even relatively low probabilities of disease are worrisome because of the seriousness of the disease. For example it would not be appropriate to send a patient with chest pain home who had a 49% probability of having acute ischemia. For this reason, models predicting acute ischemia choose a much lower cutoff, such as 7% for computing sensitivity and specificity.[67]

Another useful measure of how well your logistic regression model predicts outcome is the c index.[68] It is a measure of the concordance between predicted and observed outcomes. Here's how it works. In any data set there will be pairs of subjects who have the same observed outcome (e.g., both have had heart attacks, neither have had heart attacks) and some who have different outcomes (e.g., one had a heart attack, one did not). For all possible pairs of subjects with different outcomes, one can ask whether the model predicts a higher likelihood of outcome for the subject in the pair who experiences the outcome or for the subject who does not experience the outcome. If the subject with the higher predicted likelihood of outcome actually experiences the outcome the pair is concordant (with outcome). If the case with the higher predicted likelihood of outcome does not have the outcome, the pair is discordant. If the model predicts the same probability of outcome for both cases, the pair is tied. The c index equals the proportion of concordant cases plus half of the ties. A value of 0.5 would indicate that the model does not discriminate any better than chance. The higher the c value is (maximum 1) the greater the ability of your model to predict outcome.

---

[67] Goldman, L., Cook, E.F., Brand, D.A., et al. "A computer protocol to predict myocardial infarction in emergency department patients with chest pain." *N. Engl. J. Med.* 1988;318:797–803.

[68] Harrell, F.E., Lee, K.L., Matchar, D.B., Reichert, T.A. "Regression models for prognostic prediction: Advantages, problems, and suggested solutions." *Cancer Treat. Rep.* 1985;69:1071–77.

TABLE 9.4
Interpretation of regression coefficients.

	Multiple linear regression	Multiple logistic regression	Proportional hazards analysis
Coefficient is positive	Average value of outcome increases as independent variable increases	The logit of the outcome increases with increases in the independent variable	The logarithm of the relative hazard increases with increases in the independent variable
Coefficient is negative	Average value of outcome decreases as independent variable increases	The logit of the outcome decreases with increases in the independent variable	The logarithm of the relative hazard decreases with increases in the independent variable

9.3 What do the coefficients tell me about the relationship between each variable and the outcome?

In all three types of models, a variable's coefficient (also called beta) tells you how the outcome changes with changes in the independent variable, while adjusting for the other independent variables in the model. Coefficients can be positive or negative. Because the three different models have different types of outcome variables, there are differences in how these coefficients are interpreted (Table 9.4).

> **⯈ DEFINITION**
>
> A variable's *coefficient* tells you how the outcome changes with changes in the independent variable.

In multiple linear regression, the dependent variable is interval. This gives the coefficient a special property: It is the slope of the line describing the dependent variable. For example, let's assume that you are interested in the association between the independent variable, age (measured in years), and the outcome variable, cholesterol level (measured in mg/dl), and the coefficient for age is 0.2. The units for the coefficient would be mg/dl/year. This would mean that for each year the cholesterol increases by 0.2 mg/dl. To draw a line showing the best estimated value for all possible values of your dependent variable, all you need is the slope and a point on the y axis (where x is zero). This point is provided in linear regression by the intercept (which you will find on your printout).

With linear regression, a positive coefficient indicates that the independent variable and the outcome variable are moving (up or down) together. A negative coefficient indicates that the independent variable and the dependent variable are moving in opposite directions. So, if the coefficient is positive then the independent variable increases (e.g., age goes from 20 years to 30 years) as the average value of the outcome increases (e.g., cholesterol goes from 200 to 220 mg/dl). Conversely, a negative coefficient indicates that as the independent variable increases (e.g., age goes from 20 years to 30 years), the average value of the outcome decreases (e.g., cholesterol goes from 200 to 180 mg/dl).

The meaning of the coefficient in logistic regression is somewhat different from its meaning in linear regression. The coefficient tells you how a one-unit change in the independent variable changes the logit, which you will remember is the natural logarithm of the odds of the outcome (Section 5.2). A positive coefficient means that as the variable increases, the logit increases. A negative coefficient means that as the variable increases, the logit decreases.

To interpret the meaning of the coefficients in logistic regression, you must know which value of the outcome the logit is estimating. The default on most software programs is to determine the logit for the lower numerical value (determined by how you have coded your variables). But you could ask the computer to determine the logit of the higher numerical value. Either way, the results would be the same but the signs of the coefficients would be different. Make sure you know for which value of your outcome variable the computer is estimating the logit.

In proportional hazards analysis, the coefficients tell you how much a one-unit change in the independent variable changes the logarithm of the relative hazard. The relative hazard is the ratio of time to outcome given a particular set of risk factors to time to outcome without these factors (Section 5.2).

The meaning of the signs of the coefficients in proportional hazards analysis is similar to that in logistic regression. A positive coefficient indicates that as the independent variable increases, the logarithm of the relative hazard increases. A negative coefficient indicates that as the independent variable increases, the logarithm of the relative hazard decreases.

9.4 How do I get odds ratios and relative hazards from the multivariable analysis? What do they mean?

The coefficients in logistic regression and proportional hazards analysis have a special value. If you take the antilogarithm of the coefficient,

INTERPRETING THE ANALYSIS

you will obtain the odds ratio (for logistic regression) and the relative hazard (for proportional hazards analysis). This is simply the mathematical constant e raised to the power of the coefficient's value:

$$\text{odds ratio or relative hazard} = e^{\text{coefficient}}$$

For logistic regression the odds ratio tells you how much the likelihood of the outcome changes with a one-unit change in the independent variable. For proportional hazards analysis, the relative hazard tells you how much the time to outcome changes with a one-unit change in the independent variable. Odds ratios and relative hazards of "1" indicate that there is no change in outcome with changes in the independent variable; values greater than 1 indicate an increase in risk of outcome, while values less than 1 indicate a decrease in risk.

In published work, you will see many other terms used for the odds ratio and the relative hazard. For odds ratio, you will see relative risk, risk, and risk ratio. For relative hazard, you will see all of the terms mentioned for odds ratio plus hazard ratio and rate ratio. Odds ratio (for logistic regression) and relative hazard (for proportional hazards analysis) are the preferred terms because they distinguish results from these two types of analysis. Both the odds ratio and the relative hazard can be considered approximations of the relative risk when the outcome is rare (<15%).

The coefficients in Table 9.5 below are from a hypothetical logistic regression analysis (first column) and from an equally hypothetical proportional hazards analysis (third column). The outcome for the logistic regression analysis is heart attack at three years; the outcome for the proportional hazards analysis is time to heart attack. The coefficient for the variable history of hypertension is 0.693 in both analyses. If you take 0.693 to the e you get 2.0, meaning an odds ratio of 2.0 and a relative hazard of 2.0. (To get 2.0 enter 0.693 in your calculator, and press the button with the little e on it. If your calculator has no e bottom, buy a new calculator.)

What do these results mean? For the logistic regression analysis, it means that persons with hypertension are twice as likely as nonhypertensive persons to have a heart attack at three years. For proportional hazards analysis, it means that persons with hypertension are twice as likely to have a heart attack during the three-year study period than persons without hypertension. Note how similar these computations and interpretations are between logistic regression and proportional hazards analysis.

TABLE 9.5

Computing odds ratios and relative hazards.

	Multiple logistic regression coefficient	Odds Ratio	Proportional hazards analysis coefficient	Relative Hazard
Hypertension (yes/no)	0.693	2.0	0.693	2.0
Female gender (yes/no)	−0.693	0.5	−0.693	0.5
Age (in years)	0.182	1.2	0.182	1.2

Let's look at the next variable, female gender. It has a negative coefficient. The odds ratio is 0.5. What does this mean? It means that women are half as likely as men to have a heart attack at three years (logistic regression) and over the three-year study period (proportional hazards analysis).

How can you tell that it isn't men who are half as likely as women to have a heart attack? Actually, you cannot tell from Table 9.5. But you may assume (correctly) that I followed my own advice (Section 8.1) and coded 1 (presence of the condition – being female) and 0 (absence of the condition – being male). Since the coefficient is negative, it means that the outcome is less likely when the independent variable increases (from 0 to 1).

What would happen if you changed the coding of the gender variable such that 0 was for women and 1 was for men? The sign on the coefficient would change from negative to positive and the coefficient would stay the same. The odds ratio would change from 2.0 to .5. Has the meaning changed? First version: Women are half as likely as men to have heart attacks (odds ratio = 0.5). Second version: Men are twice as likely as women to have heart attacks (odds ratio = 2.0). The meaning is the same.

I took you through the example of gender in some detail for two reasons. First, I wanted to illustrate that the sign of the coefficient tells you whether the odds ratio will be >1 (positive sign) or <1 (negative sign). Second, I wanted you to see that you could change the coding of your dichotomous variable without changing the meaning of the analysis. Finally, I wanted to warn you how easy it is to misinterpret your results if you forget how you have coded your variables.

At the risk of public embarrassment, I will admit to you that I once completed a manuscript and circulated it to my coauthors before realizing that I had confused the coding of my variable. My finding was the opposite of what I reported in the draft of the paper. Fortunately, I found the mistake before I submitted the manuscript for publication. The reason I made the mistake (and I have seen this in other people's work as well) was that I saw what I wanted to see.

I was analyzing data on the predictors of receipt of mental health treatment among depressed persons with HIV disease.[69] I assumed that unemployment would be associated with being less likely to receive mental health services (because people wouldn't have the money to pay for treatment). Therefore, when I saw that the odds ratio for employment was 0.6, it made sense to me. It was only while performing additional analyses that I realized I had coded employment as 1 and unemployment as 0. My outcome was coded as mental health services received (1) and no mental health services received (0). My model was estimating the likelihood of receiving mental health services. Therefore, employment was associated with a decreased likelihood of receiving mental health services. It may be that employed persons receive fewer mental health services because they are less likely to be recognized as depressed by their clinicians or themselves (since they are working) or because of greater concerns of confidentiality.

You can see in Table 9.6 that for a dichotomous independent variable and a dichotomous outcome there are actually four possible codings. The results all mean the same statistically, but if you become confused (as I did) as to how you coded your variables, you can report the wrong finding.

Researchers rarely report in their manuscripts how they have coded their variables. Thus it is unlikely that a miscoded variable will be discovered in peer review. It is up to you to make sure you are reporting your results correctly.

Besides reviewing your work carefully, there are other strategies for minimizing the chance of reporting a result opposite to what your data show. First, name your variables as specifically as you can within the limits of what your statistical packages will allow (usually up to eight

✓ TIP

Name your variables as specifically as you can.

[69] Katz, M.H., Douglas, J.M., Bolan, G.A., et al. "Depression and use of mental health services among HIV-infected men." *AIDS Care* 1996;8:433–42.

TABLE 9.6

Coding of a dichotomous independent variable and outcome.

Possible coding #1	Possible coding #2
Unemployed = 0; Employed = 1	Unemployed = 1; Employed = 0
No treatment = 0; Treatment = 1	No treatment = 0; Treatment = 1
Possible coding #3	**Possible coding #4**
Unemployed = 0; Employed = 1	Unemployed = 1; Employed = 0
No treatment = 1; Treatment = 0	No treatment = 1; Treatment = 0

characters). For example, it is better to name your variable "femgend" than "gender."

It is also important to code your independent and dependent variables in a sensible way. As recommended in Section 8.1, code 0 as absence of the condition and 1 as presence. A variable such as "employ" should be coded as 1 for employment and 0 for unemployment. (I actually did this but still managed to become confused.) Alternatively, create a variable called "unemploy" and code it as 1 for unemployment and 0 for employment.

Another useful strategy is to use value labels. The computer will print out the values you have assigned each time you use the variables in the analysis. You are less likely to make a mistake if you see on your print out "1 = employment, 0 = unemployment" next to the variable. Entering value labels takes a bit of extra time at the start of your analysis, but it is worth the effort.

9.5   How do I interpret the odds ratio and relative hazard when the independent variable is interval?

Look back at Table 9.5. The variable under female gender is age. Age is an interval variable measured in years. If you take the coefficient (0.182) to the *e*, you will see that the odds ratio and relative hazards are 1.2. What does this mean? It means that, for every increase of one year in age, the likelihood of having a heart attack increases by a factor of 1.2. What would the odds ratio or relative hazard be if you coded your variable age in five-year blocks (ages 20–24, 25–29, 30–35, etc.), as many researchers do? It would be 2.5. Does it surprise you that the odds ratio and relative hazard change so much by changing the unit of measurement? Does this large change in odds ratio change the interpretation any? No. If a one-year change in age increases the risk by 1.2, then a five-year change will increase the risk by (1.2 × 1.2 × 1.2 × 1.2 × 1.2) = 2.5.

The take-home lesson here is: You cannot evaluate the importance of an odds ratio or relative hazard for an interval variable without knowing what units the independent variable is measured in. This comes up often with variables such as age and blood pressure, where a single unit change may be associated with an odds ratio or relative hazard very close to 1 (e.g., 1.2), but yet the variable has a large effect on outcome (when considered over the range of values for that independent variable).

9.6 How do I compute the confidence intervals for the odds ratios and relative hazards?

Confidence intervals tell you the range of plausible values for odds ratios and for relative hazards. They also give you a measure of the precision of your values. Large confidence intervals suggest that your sample size is insufficient for the analysis you are performing (Section 7.2).

The 95% confidence interval for the odds ratio and the relative hazard are easily obtained by extension of the formula for computing the odds ratio and relative hazard. Most statistical packages will automatically compute the confidence intervals, but some don't, and it is handy to know how to calculate it, in case you ever need to. To obtain the upper confidence interval use the addition sign; to obtain the lower confidence interval use the subtraction sign. The standard error is usually next to the coefficient on the computer printout.

$$\text{95\% confidence interval for odds ratio/relative hazard} = e^{\text{coefficient} \pm 1.96(\text{standard error})}$$

Looking at the formula you can also see how the precision of your estimate (measured by the standard error) is reflected in the confidence intervals. If the standard error is large you will be adding (or subtracting) a large number from the coefficient. This will result in the upper limit being much bigger than the odds ratio/relative hazard and the lower limit being much smaller than the odds ratio/relative hazard.

Of course, you don't have to use 95% confidence intervals. For some exploratory studies you may wish to report 90% confidence intervals. For other studies, where precision is very important, you may wish to report 99% confidence intervals. The formula is the same as the one shown above except that instead of 1.96, which is the standard normal deviate for 95% confidence intervals, you substitute the standard normal deviate for the confidence intervals you want (1.66 for 90% confidence intervals; 2.576 for 99% confidence intervals.)

9.7 What are standardized coefficients and should I use them?

Standardized regression coefficients are your regression coefficients multiplied by the standard deviation for that independent variable and divided by the standard deviation of the dependent variable:

$$\text{standardized regression coefficient} = \text{regression coefficient} \times \frac{\text{standard deviation of independent variable}}{\text{standard deviation of dependent variable}}$$

> **✓ TIP**
>
> To compare the magnitude of coefficients of independent variables that are measured on different scales, standardize them.

Unless you standardize your coefficients you cannot compare the magnitude of coefficients of independent variables that are measured on different scales. If you divide your independent variable by ten (e.g., switch from age in years to age in decades), it will increase your coefficient by ten. Obviously dividing a variable by ten does not in any way change the association between that variable and the outcome. However, if you divide the variable by ten, not only will the coefficient increase tenfold, so will the standard deviation. By multiplying the coefficient by the ratio of the two standard deviations, the coefficient becomes unitless (the units cancel each other out). You can therefore compare across different independent variables because they are all on the same scale. Of course, if all of your independent variables are on the same scale, as will be true if all your variables are dichotomous, then standardization is unnecessary. The downside of standardized coefficients is that you lose a sense of the actual effect (in real units) that each variable has on the dependent variable.

The above formula works for both multiple linear regression and logistic regression. The only difference is that the standard deviation

INTERPRETING THE ANALYSIS

of the dependent variable in logistic regression is not a calculated value but is the constant 1.81. With multiple linear regression, the square of the standardized coefficient also gives you a sense of the proportion of variance explained by that variable (like a partial R^2). This is not true with logistic regression. Standardized coefficients are rarely reported with proportional hazards models.[70]

9.8 How do I test the statistical significance of my coefficients?

The smart answer to this question is that you read the P value next to the variable on the printout. Although this is perfectly true, it is worth understanding where these P values come from.

If you understand the difference between unstandardized and standardized regression coefficients (Section 9.7), then you know that you cannot judge the strength of the association between an independent variable and an outcome by the size of the coefficient (because the size is determined by the size of your units). But you can eyeball whether a coefficient is significant by looking at the unstandardized coefficient and the standard error of the coefficient. How?

Well, remember that a statistical model only *estimates* the true value of the parameter in the population you are studying. There is an error associated with that estimate (the standard error). Common sense tells you that if the size of the standard error is similar to the (absolute) size of the coefficient (the error is as big as the effect), the effect won't be significant.

However, if the coefficient is much bigger than the standard error, the coefficient may be statistically significant. Look at Table 9.7. The coefficients and the standard errors are from the study of factors associated with receipt of PCP prophylaxis (Section 7.1). Without looking back at the discussion of the study results, can you tell which of the variables are statistically significant?

If you said the variables nonwhite ethnicity and no insurance, you are right. You can tell because the standard errors for these variables are much smaller than the coefficient for these variables. Note that the coefficient is larger for the variable gay men than for the variables nonwhite ethnicity and no insurance. Yet this variable is not significant because the coefficient is not large relative to its standard error.

---

[70] For more on standardized coefficients see Feinstein, A.R. *Multivariable Analysis: An Introduction*. New Haven: Yale University Press, 1996, pp. 222–5, 322, 330, 391.

Also note that I did not need to remind you that these coefficients were from logistic regression. That's because it doesn't really matter. With any of the three multivariable techniques, a coefficient that is more that twice the size of the standard error is likely to be statistically significant. In Table 9.8, I have included the P values as well as the odds ratios and the confidence intervals.

Some other points are worth noting from Table 9.8. In Section 7.1, I pointed out that because of the small number of women in this study, the confidence intervals for the odds ratio for the gender variable were very large. You can see this just by looking at the coefficient and the standard error. Note that the standard error is about six times the size of the coefficient. It stands to reason that if the error is bigger than the effect, the effect cannot be a very reliable estimate. You can also see that the two variables that are statistically significant are also the ones where the confidence intervals for the odds ratios exclude 1. This should serve as a reminder to you that confidence intervals depend on similar assumptions as P values (i.e., the size of the effect compared to the size of the error).

The methods for computing the P values are similar for linear regression, logistic regression, and proportional hazards analysis. For

> **✓ T I P**
>
> If the error is bigger than the effect, the effect cannot be a very reliable estimate.

TABLE 9.8
Coefficients, standard errors, P values, and confidence intervals for receipt of PCP prophylaxis.

Variable	Coefficient	Standard error	P value	Odds ratio	Upper 95% confidence interval	Lower 95% confidence interval
Age ≤35 years	.1696	.2846	.55	1.19	.68	2.07
Nonwhite ethnicity	−.7173	.2922	.01	.49	.28	.87
Male gender	−.2162	1.2910	.87	.81	.06	10.12
Gay men	1.1592	.7183	.11	3.19	.78	13.03
Injection drug users	.1068	.4221	.80	1.11	.49	2.55
No insurance	−1.0356	.3656	.005	.35	.17	.73

Adopted with permission from Schwarcz, S.K., et al. "Prevention of *Pneumocystis carinii* pneumonia: Who are we missing?" *AIDS* 1997;11:1263–68. Copyright Rapid Science Publishers Ltd. Additional data supplied by the authors.

multiple linear regression, the P value is based on a t test, where t is

$$t = \frac{\text{coefficient}}{\text{standard error}}$$

You can determine the significance of t, if you know the degrees of freedom (sample size − the number of parameters, where the parameters are the independent variables plus the intercept). You can then look up the significance of the t value in the tables that are at the back of most standard statistical books (but not this one). More likely you will read it off your printout. But, of interest, t values greater than 2.0 (coefficient is two times the standard error) are statistically significant at the traditional $P < .05$ value (as long as the degrees of freedom are at least sixty).

Logistic regression and proportional hazards analysis use a similar test, called the Wald test, for determining the importance of an individual coefficient. It is based on either the chi-squared or the z distribution:

$$\text{chi-squared distribution} = \left\{ \frac{\text{coefficient}}{\text{standard error}} \right\}^2 \quad \text{or} \quad z \text{ distribution} = \frac{\text{coefficient}}{\text{standard error}}$$

With either formula, coefficients that are twice their standard error

> **✓ TIP**
> Use the Wald chi-square for testing the significance of individual coefficients.

will be significant at $P < .05$. The Wald test assumes a large sample size (i.e., 80–100 or more subjects).

For logistic regression and proportional hazards analysis there are two other tests that you can use to determine the statistical significance of a particular coefficient: the likelihood ratio statistic and the score test.[71] The likelihood ratio test is based on comparing the likelihood when the variable is not in the model to the likelihood when the variable is in the model. To compute the statistic for models where you have multiple independent variables, each variable is singly dropped while retaining the other variables in the model. The statistic follows a chi-squared distribution. Computation of the score test is based on derivatives of the likelihood ratio. It also follows a chi-squared distribution.

Although there are situations when the likelihood ratio test may perform better,[72] most researchers use the Wald chi-square. If your results are robust you should get similar results with all three tests.

9.9 How do I interpret the results of interaction terms?

Having reviewed the meaning of coefficients, let's return to the question of how to interpret product terms used to represent interaction effects (Section 8.3). If the impact of the two variables together is substantially greater than the additive effect of the two variables, the coefficient will be positive and statistically significant. If the impact of the two variables together is substantially less then the additive effect of the two variables, the coefficient will be negative and statistically significant.

9.10 Do I have to adjust my multivariable regression coefficients for multiple comparisons?

When you perform multiple bivariate comparisons (for example, comparing two groups on twenty different variables), some statisticians

---

[71] You met the likelihood ratio test in Section 9.2.A on evaluating whether your model accounts for outcome better than chance. The difference is that here you are comparing models with a particular variable present to models where that variable is absent (but the other independent variables are present). In Section 9.2.A this test compared models that contained all of the independent variables to models that contained none of the independent variables.

[72] Hauck, W.W., Donner, A. "Wald's test as applied to hypotheses in logit analysis." *J. Am. Stat. Assoc.* 72:851–53.

recommend adjusting for multiple comparisons. The theory is that, by chance, at least one of your twenty comparisons will be statistically significant at the $P < .05$ level (that's because $1/20 = .05$). With multivariable analysis, you need not worry about multiple comparisons when performing tests of the significance of the overall model (F or likelihood ratio test). The reason is that you are performing only a single test to assess whether the independent variables (as a group) are associated with the outcome without worrying about adjusting for multiple comparisons.

But when you turn to the question of whether the individual independent variables from your multivariable model are statistically associated with your outcome, you are essentially making multiple comparisons. As with bivariate comparisons, some statisticians advocate adjusting your P value for the number of independent variables in your model. The most common and easiest method is the Bonferoni correction. It "charges" you for the number of independent variables in the model by requiring a lower P value before concluding that a comparison is statistically significant. To calculate the correction simply divide the usual P value (e.g., .05) by the number of variables in the model. If you have ten variables, you would require that the P value be $<.005$ ($.05/10$) before concluding that the association between the independent variable and the outcome is significant.

DEFINITION

The *Bonferoni correction* "charges" you for the number of independent variables in the model by requiring a lower *P* value before concluding that a comparison is statistically significant.

There are major disadvantages to adjusting for multiple comparisons. They have been well articulated by the epidemiologist Kenneth Rothman.[73] He points out that the basis of adjustment for multiple comparisons is the assumption that chance is the most common explanation for an association between two things. But this assumption is flawed because the universe is governed by natural (physical) laws. Most associations in the universe have a true (rather than chance) connection. (Note that a true connection does not mean a causal connection.)

In addition, an individual comparison cannot "know" how many other comparisons you have made. Therefore an individual association cannot be more or less likely due to chance based on how many other associations you have assessed. Rothman illustrates the absurdity of strict adherence to the principle of adjusting for multiple comparisons by asking: If you favor adjusting for multiple comparisons, should you adjust for the number of comparisons you assessed in a single paper,

[73] Rothman, K.J. "No adjustments are needed for multiple comparisons." *Epidemiology* 1990;1:43–6.

or the number of comparisons assessed in a series of papers analyzing the same data set, or number of the comparisons performed during your career?

Personally, I am swayed by Rothman's arguments and do not adjust for multiple comparisons. Nonetheless, if you are not going to adjust for multiple comparisons, there are measures that you should take to minimize potential problems. Tell your reader how many variables (comparisons) were tested in your analysis. Do not report only the independent variables that were significantly associated with outcome. Nonsignificant results, while much less sexy, are every bit as informative. Do not be a slave to the cutoff of $P < .05$, in either direction. Don't assume something is insignificant just because its P value is .06 or that something is significant just because its P value is .04. Use confidence intervals, whenever possible, instead of P values (although, as discussed above, confidence intervals are also subject to the potential multiple comparison problem, since they are based on the 95% probability that the true value falls within the interval). Most importantly, evaluate your findings in light of previous work and biological plausibility. If you anticipate that a reviewer will not be convinced by the above, cite Rothman's article. It sometimes helps.[74]

✓ **T I P**

To minimize potential problems with multiple comparisons, tell your reader how many variables were tested in your analysis, report significant and nonsignificant results, and don't be a slave to the cutoff of $P < .05$.

[74] For more on the debate about multiple comparisons, see: Savitz, D.A., Olshan, A.F. "Multiple comparisons and related issues in the interpretation of epidemiologic data." *Am. J. Epidemiol.* 1995;142:904–8; Thompson, J. "Re: 'Multiple comparisons and related issues in the interpretation of epidemiologic data.'" *Am. J. Epidemiol.* 1997;147:801–6; Goodman, S.N. "Multiple comparisons, explained." *Am. J. Epidemiol.* 1997;147:807–12; Savitz, D.A., Olshan, A.F. "Describing data requires no adjustment for multiple comparisons: A reply from Savitz and Olshan." *Am. J. Epidemiol.* 1997;147:813–14; Thompson, J.R. "A response to 'Describing data requires no adjustment for multiple comparisons.'" *Am. J. Epidemiol.* 1997;147:815.

INTERPRETING THE ANALYSIS

10

Checking the Assumptions of the Analysis

10.1 How do I know if my data fit the assumptions of my multivariable model?

In Chapter 5, we reviewed the ways to assess, in bivariate analysis, whether the relationship between a single independent variable and outcome fit the assumptions of your model. In this chapter, we will review how to assess whether these assumptions are fulfilled on a multivariable level.

For didactic purposes, I have separated the discussion of whether your data fit the assumptions of your model from the discussion of how well your model accounts for the outcome (Section 9.2). But, in fact, these two topics are closely related. In a model where your independent variables closely account for your outcome, it is likely that your data fit the assumptions of your model. Conversely, if your model does not appear to fit your observed outcome, the reason might be that your data do not fit the assumptions of the model. When this is the case, adding, deleting, or transforming variables may improve the fit of your model. Part of why I separated the discussion of these two issues is that most researchers will interpret their multivariable printouts, make changes, and add or delete variables before going on to verify the assumptions of their final model.

Residual analysis is a helpful tool for assessing whether your data fit the assumptions of your multivariable model. Residuals are the difference between the observed and the estimated value. They can be thought of as the error in estimation. A good model will have most residuals close to 0, meaning that the observed and estimated values are close to one another. When the observed is greater than the estimated value the residual is positive; when the observed value is less, the residual is negative.

⫸ DEFINITION

Residuals are the difference between the observed and the estimated value.

141

Besides helping you to test if your data fit the assumptions of your model, residual analysis can also help you to identify individual subjects whose values on the outcome variable do not fit with the other subjects (outliers).

Residual analysis is more art than science.

I mention in passing that while residual analysis is valuable it is more art than science. You may get alarming patterns of residuals even though your data fit the assumptions of your model. It is also possible for your residuals to look fine, and yet your data do not fit the assumptions of your model. Small samples are especially likely to yield messy residuals. With large samples, multivariable models are sufficiently robust that departures from the assumptions of the model, seen on residual analysis, are unlikely to cause significant problems.

10.2 How do I assess the linearity, normal distribution, and equal variance assumptions of multiple linear regression?

Linear regression assumes linearity, normal distribution, and equal variance around the mean (Chapter 5). To test whether your interval-independent variables fit a linear relationship with outcome in your multivariable model, plot your residuals against your independent variables and the estimated outcome variable. If the relationship is linear, the points will be symmetric above and below a straight line, with roughly equal spread along the line. In contrast, if residuals are particularly large at very high and/or low levels of one of the independent variables or estimated dependent variable, it suggests a significant departure from linearity.[75]

Plots of residuals against any of the independent variables and the estimated dependent variable also demonstrate whether your model fulfills the assumptions of normal distribution and equal variance. When these assumptions are met the residuals should be close to zero and the spread of values should be equal both above and below zero. If, instead, the residuals are far from zero and there is not equal spread of values above and below zero (e.g., a few of the residual points are far from the zero line indicating outliers) the assumptions of normal distribution and equal variance are not met.

[75] For a detailed description of analysis of residuals including numerous graphs see Glantz, S.A., Slinker, B.K. *Primer of Applied Regression and Analysis of Variance.* New York: McGraw-Hill, 1990, pp. 110–80.

Besides plotting the residuals against the independent variable or the estimated dependent variable, it is also possible to test the assumptions of multivariable normal distribution by plotting standardized residuals on a normal probability plot. If the residuals are normally distributed with equal variance the plot will appear as a straight line. If, instead, you see a nonlinear pattern, such as an S-shape, this suggests that the assumptions of normal distribution are not fulfilled. Points far from the line indicate outliers.

If your plots do not fit the assumptions of linear regression, don't give up. Look back in the section on transforming variables (Sections 5.5 and 5.8). It may be that by transforming one of your independent or dependent variables you will achieve a better model. Also, if your sample size is greater than 100, you can assume that the assumption of normal distribution is met for your independent variables (Section 5.7).

10.3 How do I assess the linearity assumption of multiple logistic regression and proportional hazards analysis?

As with multiple linear regression, residual analysis can help you determine if your interval-independent variables show a linear relationship with outcome. To do this, plot your residuals or standardized residuals against the independent variable. If the linear assumption is met, the residuals should be about the same for all values of your independent variable. Larger residuals as the independent variable gets larger (or smaller or both) suggests that your model does not fit the linear assumption.

Another method of assessing the linear assumption of interval variables is to create multiple dichotomous variables of equal intervals of your variable. I explained this technique in Section 5.4. The only difference here is that you will be using it to assess whether your independent variable fits the linearity assumption after adjustment for other independent variables. If the numeric difference between the coefficients of each successive group is approximately equal, this is consistent with a linear gradient.

Finally, some researchers will assess whether an interval variable has a linear gradient by substituting a transformed version of the variable for the variable itself. Commonly, logarithmic and quadratic transformations are tested. If the coefficient for that variable increases and the fit of the model improves with the transformation, this would suggest that the variable more closely fits a logarithmic or quadratic gradient.

You should be aware that with logistic regression you may get extremely disturbing appearing residuals even if your model is sound. This is especially likely to occur when you have strong dichotomous (rather than interval) independent variables.

10.4 What are outliers and how do I detect them in my multiple linear regression models?

Outliers are points that do not follow the pattern of the other points. For example, Figure 10.1 shows a linear relationship with higher values of the independent variable associated with higher values of the outcome. While most of the points conform to this linear relationship, two points (A and B) do not fit this relationship. Point A has a much higher value for outcome than you would expect given the intermediate value on the independent variable. Point B has a much lower value of outcome than you would expect given the high value of the independent variable.

In addition to graphical presentations, outliers can be detected in linear regression by several residual measures that are calculated by most statistical packages: standardized residuals, studentized residuals, leverage, and Cook's distance.

Standardized residuals help pinpoint outliers. Standardized residuals larger than two are the extreme 5% of values, whereas those larger than three are the extreme 1% of values.

Studentized residuals adjust for how far each individual value is from the center of the line. The result is that two points an equal distance from the line will have different studentized residuals: The studentized residual will be larger for the value at the extremes of the line than the value at the center. This is because values at the extremes are likely to be influential. They can more easily tilt the line. Think of a seesaw, with the center point as the fulcrum and the extreme points as the ends of the plank. Exerting pressure on the end will cause the entire plank to change slope. Such points are referred to as leverage points and are more influential in the analysis. With studentized residuals, leverage points will get a larger residual than an outlier whose value is close to the center of the line. So in Figure 10.1 point B will have a larger studentized residual than point A even though these points are the same distance from the line. I have used a thicker dotted line in

> **✓ TIP**
>
> Outliers at the extremes of the value of the independent value are more influential than those closer to the midpoint.

CHECKING THE ASSUMPTIONS OF THE ANALYSIS

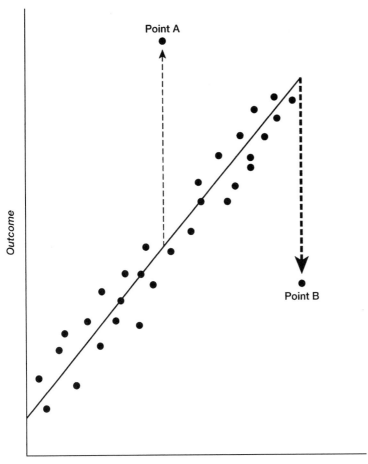

Figure 10.1. Linear relationship between an independent variable and outcome with two outliers (point A and point B). The thicker dotted line pointing to B illustrates the greater influence of point B compared to point A.

Figure 10.1 to point to B to illustrate the greater influence of point B compared to point A.

The measure leverage quantifies the influence of individual points on the line. Ideally, all your observations should have leverage measures less than two times the expected value. The expected value is the number of variables +1 divided by the sample size. Cook's distance offers another way of telling how influential an individual point is on the overall model. It is equal to the change in the regression coefficients if the observation was deleted.

10.5   How do I detect outliers in my multiple logistic regression model?

Many of the same statistics that detect outliers in multiple linear regression are available for multiple logistic regression, including raw residuals, standardized residuals, studentized residuals, leverage, and Cook's distance. In addition, the Pearson and deviance residuals are also particularly useful for assessing multiple logistic regression models.

As with linear regression, standardized or studentized residuals greater than 2–3 suggest outliers. Subjects with leverage values exceeding twice the expected value (number of independent variables divided by the sample size) are very influential. Cook's value greater than 1 also suggests a point of heavy influence.

A helpful test both for assessing outliers as well as the overall fit of the model is to plot the Pearson and deviance residual against the estimated probability of outcome. This will show you whether the model is less successful in estimating outcome at particular probabilities.[76]

10.6   What about analysis of residuals with proportional hazards analysis?

Residual analysis is rarely used with proportional hazards analysis. Readers interested in learning more about their use should see Kalbfleisch and Prentice.[77]

10.7   What should I do when I detect outliers?

Let's say that your analysis of residuals suggests you have certain extreme values. What do you do? First, check to make sure there is no error in the recording of this data point. You may think that this is an unnecessary step if you have already reviewed your univariate results for extreme values (Section 5.7). But review of outliers from multivariable analysis complements the univariate analysis. For example, residual analysis of a multivariable model may detect an obese diabetic

---

[76] For a detailed review of residuals with logistic regression see Hosmer, D.W, Lemeshow, S. *Applied Logistic Regression*. New York: Wiley, 1989, pp. 149–70.

[77] See Kalbfleisch, J.D., Prentice, R.L. *The Statistical Analysis of Failure Time Data*. New York: Wiley, 1980, pp. 96–8.

with a heavy fat consumption whose cholesterol is abnormally low (140 mg/dl). This may result in your discovering a data entry error: The value was really 410 mg/dl. Since a cholesterol level of 140 mg/dl is not an extreme value you would not have noticed a problem in the univariate analysis.

But what if you verify from the original data that this subject's value really is 140 mg/dl? Do you delete it from the data set? No. If you were performing a laboratory experiment, and had a residual value that did not fit your analysis, you might want to repeat the experiment. But in clinical trials this is rarely an option. While it may be tempting to delete such values from the study (especially if they are preventing you from getting the answer you were hoping for) this is rarely justified. Just because certain subjects are outliers, it doesn't mean their values are wrong. In fact, it is "normal" to have a few extreme values.

However, if your residuals indicate leverage points you may want to consider removing them from the analysis, repeating the analysis, and seeing whether your findings hold. If deletion of a couple of observations changes your entire analysis, the analysis may not be valid. In general, the larger your data set is, the less likely it is that your results will be heavily influenced by one or two points. Therefore, the need to closely examine the residuals of all of your points becomes less important.

10.8 What is the additive assumption and how do I assess whether my multiple independent variables fit this assumption?

All three multivariable models assume that your multiple independent variables have an additive effect on the outcome.

In the case of multiple linear regression, the change in the mean value of the outcome is modeled as the sum of the individual effects of the independent variables on outcome (Section 5.3). While both logistic regression and proportional hazards analysis have the same additive assumption, it is more confusing with these two techniques because with logistic regression and proportional hazards analysis we are not modeling the outcome itself. Rather we are modeling the logit of the outcome and the logarithm of the relative hazard, respectively.

With logistic regression, the logit of the outcome is modeled as the sum of the individual independent variables. With proportional hazards analysis, the logarithm of the relative hazard is modeled as

> ✓ **TIP**
>
> The effect of multiple variables on the odds ratio or the relative hazard is multiplicative.

the sum of the individual independent variables. The consequence of this is that the odds ratio or relative hazard for the effect of multiple variables on outcome is multiplicative, rather than additive. Statisticians refer to this with the somewhat confusing term of "additive on a multiplicative scale."

Although I didn't refer to it as the additive assumption, we have dealt with this concept in the discussion of interactions (Sections 1.4, 8.3, and 9.9). Interactions are present when the variables are not additive but rather something greater or less than additive.

If you look back at the discussion of the interaction of gender and ST elevations shown in Section 1.4, you see that I multiplied the odds ratios to show the meaning of the interaction. Specifically, in Table 1.7, the odds ratio for male gender was 1.6 and the odds ratio for ST elevations was 8.1. Since the model is "additive on a multiplicative scale" the odds ratio associated with being male and having ST elevations should be the product of the two or $13.0 (1.6 \times 8.1 = 13.0)$.

But the risk of heart attack for men with ST elevations was not 13 times the risk for women without ST elevations. How do we know this? Because the product term was statistically significant. To find out the true risk for men with ST elevations, you need to include the interaction term, which had an odds ratio of 0.6. When you include the product term you learn that the risk for men with ST elevations is less than 13.0; it is actually only $7.8 (1.6 \times 8.1 \times 0.6 = 7.8)$. After reading Section 9.9, you would have known that the overall risk would have been lower just from the negative sign of the coefficient of the product term.

What does all this mean? Clinically, as discussed in Section 1.4, it means that the difference in the likelihood of heart attacks between men and women vanishes in the presence of ST elevations. (The risk for women with ST elevations is $8.1(1.0 \times 8.1 \times 1.0 = 8.1)$, essentially identical to the risk of 7.8 in men with ST elevations $(1.6 \times 8.1 \times 0.6 = 7.8)$. In terms of your model, this means that in the absence of including an interaction term for gender and ST elevations, your model would have been misspecified because the additive assumption would not have been fulfilled.

You may be asking yourself, why does the model without interaction terms estimate that men with ST elevations have a significantly higher risk of heart attack than women with ST elevations, if the risk for these two groups is similar? To understand why remember that each variable (e.g., gender, ST elevations) has only one coefficient. Therefore, the best coefficient for the sample as a whole may not be best for

---

✓ **T I P**

The best coefficient for the sample as a whole may not be best for every subgroup of subjects.

CHECKING THE ASSUMPTIONS OF THE ANALYSIS

every subgroup of subjects as defined by the independent variables. In other words, just because men have a greater risk of heart attack than women and persons with ST elevations have a greater risk than persons without ST elevations does not mean that men with ST elevations have a greater risk than women with ST elevations. This illustrates how models without product terms can be wrong for particular subsets of subjects. Product terms solve this problem by having another variable that can improve the fit of the model for particular subgroups of subjects.

Assessing whether your variables fulfill the additive assumption becomes especially complicated when you realize that in most analyses there are a large number of possible interactions terms. For example there are forty-five possible two-way interactions between just ten independent variables. And there is nothing to prevent interactions from being three-way (e.g., male × ST elevations × prior heart attack). Short of trying all possible product terms, there is no way to know for certain if your data contain an important interaction.

One clue that you may need an interaction term is that a variable that you thought, based on clinical grounds, would have an important effect on an outcome variable did not. Could it be that the variable is important only under certain conditions? Other clues may come from your analysis of how well your data fit the assumptions of your model. For example, if the standardized residuals do not form a straight line on the normal probability plot or if your logistic regression residuals are particularly large, the reason may be that you have an interaction.

Besides the fact that interactions are difficult to detect there are other problems. Some statistically significant interactions are very difficult to interpret clinically. In addition, if you test a large number of interactions, it is likely that at least one of them will be statistically significant. Does that mean that this is an important interaction?

In this regard, testing for interaction is similar to performing subgroup analysis. Let's say that a study finds that a new drug is no better than placebo in the sample as a whole. However, when the investigators looked within ten subgroups, they found one group (e.g., hypertensive women with diabetes) for whom the drug worked. Would you conclude that the drug works for hypertensive women with diabetes?

In general, unless there is some reason to believe that the drug should work only in hypertensive women with diabetes, and the authors had therefore planned this subgroup analysis, one would conclude that the drug does not work and the finding was chance. That is, in some subgroups, the drug worked better than placebo. In other subgroups, the drug worked worse than placebo. Overall, there was no effect. The same issue exists if you test ten product terms. If the main effect is null, and nine of the product terms are insignificant, and one of them is significant, do you conclude that overall the drug works in that special condition? Probably not.

Because of these problems, many clinical researchers do not test for interactions at all. In contrast, it is common in the epidemiologic literature to evaluate all possible two-way interactions. The methodological justification is that if a product term is significant, it is improving the statistical quality of the model. However, this strategy is not usually pursued in the medical literature because of the difficulty of making clinical sense out of product terms.

My own preference is to test only for those interactions that are theoretically important. That is the strategy that was pursued in the study described above of the impact of gender on heart attack risk. The researchers evaluated all possible interactions involving gender because it was known that the variables associated with heart attack are different in men and women and because this was the focus of their study. But they did not assess all possible interactions in their data set (e.g., age × race).

Whatever strategy you employ for assessing interactions, it is important to tell your reader whether and how you have tested for interactions. Depending on what strategy you have chosen, you can tell your reader that you:

- tested all primary (second-degree) interactions, or
- tested specific interactions (and detail them), or
- chose not to test any interactions.

10.9 What does the additive assumption mean for interval-independent variables?

The meaning of the additive assumption for interval-independent variables is analogous to its meaning for multiple independent variables.

For multiple linear regression the change in the mean value of the outcome (on a simple arithmetic scale) is modeled as the sum of the unit changes of the interval-independent variable. The situation is more complicated with logistic regression and proportional hazards analysis. As with multiple independent variables, changes on an interval-independent variable are "additive on a multiplicative scale." Thus, if you have an interval-independent variable, such as blood pressure, the additive assumption would mean that the odds ratio or relative hazard associated with a 20 mm increase in blood pressure would be twice the odds ratio or relative hazard associated with a 10 mm increase in blood pressure. Numerically, if the increase in risk due to a 10 mm increase of blood pressure from 140 to 149 mm is 1.4, then the increase in risk due to an increase from 140 to 159 mm is 1.96 (1.4 × 1.4).

In Section 5.4, I suggested that one way to assess the linear assumption of an interval variable was to categorize the variable into multiple categorical variables, maintaining the interval nature of the scale. This procedure allows you to see if the differences between sequential coefficients are about the same (as you would expect if the relationship is linear). As an extension of this method, you can include the other independent variables in the model and thereby assess whether the interval-independent variable fits the additive assumption with statistical adjustment for the other covariates.

10.10   What is the proportionality assumption?

The proportionality assumption is relevant only to proportional hazards analysis (Section 5.1). The assumption is that the hazards for persons with different patterns of covariates are constant over time. In other words, if the relative hazard of heart attack among diabetics is three times higher than among nondiabetics in the first year of the study, the relative hazard of heart attack must also be (about) three times higher among diabetics than nondiabetics in the second year of the study. Note that the hazard for a heart attack can be very different in the first year than in the second year (e.g., much higher in the first year than in the second year), but the difference between the hazards for diabetics and nondiabetics must be constant throughout the study period.

> **▶ DEFINITION**
>
> The *proportionality assumption* is that the hazards for persons with different patterns of covariates are constant over time.

While the proportionality assumption may, at first, sound complicated, it is really very simple. Since proportional hazards analysis, like multiple linear and logistic regression, provides you with a single coefficient for each variable, that coefficient, and its associated relative hazard, must represent the risk throughout the time period. If the risk of outcome associated with a particular variable is higher at one point in time and lower at another, a single coefficient cannot represent that relationship.

For example, in Figure 10.2 we see that the risk of death among patients with acute nonlymphoblastic leukemia is not constant over

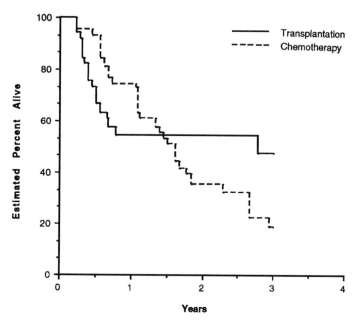

Figure 10.2. Kaplan-Meier curves show the estimated probability of survival for the chemotherapy group (broken line) and the transplantation group (solid line). Reproduced with permission from Appelbaum, F.R., et al. "Bone marrow transplantation or chemotherapy after remission induction for adults with acute nonlymphoblastic leukemia." *Ann. Intern. Med.* 1984;101:581–8.

time in the two arms of the study.[78] Patients who received a bone marrow transplant were more likely to die in the first year. But, thereafter, the risk was lower than with conventional chemotherapy.

If you used proportional hazards analysis to analyze the effect of transplantation on death, the relative hazard would likely be one. The higher risk of death associated with transplantation in the first year and a half and the lower risk of death associated with transplantation in the period between a year and a half and three years would average out. Although this average risk of one is arguably the best single estimate of the difference in risk of death with transplantation compared to chemotherapy, you would not want to tell your patients that the risk of death with the two treatments was the same. It would be more informative to tell them that bone marrow transplant is a toxic treatment and that there are a significant number of deaths due to

[78] Appelbaum, F.R., Dahlberg, S., Thomas, E.D., et al. "Bone marrow transplantation or chemotherapy after remission induction for adults with acute nonlymphoblastic leukemia." *Ann. Intern. Med.* 1984;101:581–8.

the treatment. However, if they survive the treatment, their survival at three years is significantly better than with conventional therapy.

Some researchers will assess the proportionality assumption only for the main effect in their study (e.g., treatment versus no treatment). However, if potential confounders do not meet the proportionality assumption you may not be adequately adjusting for them in the analysis. For this reason, it is important to assess whether all your variables fulfill the proportionality assumption, and not just the main effect you are studying.

10.11 How do I test the proportionality assumption?

The proportionality assumption can be assessed for a single independent variable with Kaplan–Meier survival curves. When the proportionality assumption is met, there should be a steadily increasing difference between the two curves. In contrast, if the two curves cross, as in the case of the transplantation versus chemotherapy study, the proportionality assumption is violated (Figure 10.2).

> ✓ **TIP**
>
> If the curves cross, the proportionality assumption is violated.

There are more sophisticated methods for assessing whether the proportional hazards assumption is met. Two commonly used methods are: graphical representations and time-dependent variables. The graph is referred to as a log-minus-log survival plot (Figure 10.3). If there is a constant (vertical) difference between the two curves then you know that the hazards of subjects with different values on a particular independent variable are proportional over time.

A nice feature of log-minus-log survival curves is that they illustrate that proportional hazards analysis makes no assumption about the absolute risks (the lines change direction and slope). Proportional hazards analysis only assumes that as the hazards change, the distance between the two curves stays about the same. The curves do not have to be perfectly equidistant. Especially at the ends of the curves, where there tend to be fewer observations, there may be some coming together or greater splitting of the curves. A limitation of log-minus-log survival curves is that, as with Kaplan–Meier curves, you can assess whether the proportionality assumption is fulfilled for only one variable at a time.

Another way of testing the proportionality assumption is to add interaction terms to the proportional hazards model that allow the relative hazard to vary over time. The interaction terms are called time-dependent covariates (Section 12.4); they require special coding, which varies by statistical package. They can be created so that the

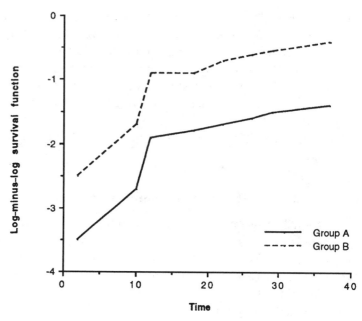

Figure 10.3. Log-minus-log survival plot showing a constant difference between group A (solid line) and group B (broken line). Reprinted with permission from Katz, M.H., Hauck, W.W. "Proportional hazards (Cox) regression." *J. Gen. Intern. Med.* 1993;8: 702–11.

logarithm of the relative hazards is allowed to vary linearly with time or with the logarithm of time. When the proportionality assumption is valid, the interaction term will have a hazard ratio near 1.0 (no effect) and will not be statistically significant. If the odds ratio is significantly different from 1.0 it means that the effect of the independent variable does vary over time (the proportionality assumption is not met).

The advantage of time-dependent covariates is that you can create more than one such term and assess simultaneously whether the proportionality assumption is met for multiple independent variables. However, if your sample size is small, you may not be able to enter interaction terms for all variables in the model simultaneously (there may be too many variables for the sample size). In that case, you can add each product term individually to your other variables to see if the product term is significant with adjustment for the other variables in the model. A potential disadvantage of time-dependent covariates is that, if your sample is really large, time interaction terms may be too sensitive. You may get statistically significant terms even though the

CHECKING THE ASSUMPTIONS OF THE ANALYSIS

graphical representation does not show a major departure from the proportionality assumption.

Alternatively, you can construct your model such that the relative hazard varies by period, taking on one value in the first X time units, another value in the next Y time units, and so on. This approach is analogous to transforming an interval-independent variable (in this case time) into a categorical variable. With this approach you can test whether the relative hazards between periods are statistically different.

For example, we were performing an analysis of the impact of socioeconomic status on survival with AIDS.[79] We assessed the proportionality assumption using log-minus-log survival curves. Most of the curves looked fine. But one of the covariates, an initial AIDS diagnosis of cryptosporidiosis, looked suspicious for violating the proportionality assumption. Because we were not sure, we tested the hypothesis. Instead of the single variable cryptosporidiosis (yes/no), we created two covariates: cryptosporidiosis in the first period of study time and cryptosporidiosis in the second period of study time (yes/no). The cutoff for the time period was chosen based on the log-minus-log survival plot (the point where it seemed the relative hazard changed).

Using proportional hazards analysis we tested the hypothesis that the two variables were significantly different from one another. The P value was only marginally significant (.07.) Although this was above the conventional cutoff of P value $<.05$, P values less than $<.20$ can indicate important changes in risk over time. However, the variable cryptosporidiosis was not the major variable of interest in our study. We were looking for the relationship between socioeconomic status and survival. Our goal was to adequately adjust for AIDS diagnoses that might confound the relationship between socioeconomic status and AIDS survival. Since we were unsure how important this potential departure from the proportionality assumption was for our study, we tested whether a proportional hazards model that included these two time period variables instead of the one covariate changed any of the other coefficients in important ways. It did not. We therefore chose to report the simpler model (to make the study more interpretable for readers), adjusting only for the variable cryptosporidiosis. We explained what we had done in the Methods section (of course!). Had it been a study focused on how cryptosporidiosis affected AIDS survival

[79] Katz, M.H., Hsu, L., Lingo, M., Woelffer, G., Schwarcz, S.K. "Impact of socioeconomic status on survival with AIDS." *Am. J. Epidemiol.* 1998;148:282–91.

and/or had the two covariates changed the coefficients of our other variables, we would have included these time period variables in the final model.

10.12 What if the proportionality assumption does not hold for my data?

You have a few choices (besides abandoning your research career!). You can divide your observation period such that within any one period the odds are proportional. If you do this, you will have two or more proportional hazards analyses. The factors associated with outcome would differ for the two periods (e.g., diabetics will have a higher risk in the model estimating heart attack during the first three months and a lower risk in the model estimating heart attack in the second three-month period).

A second strategy is to perform a stratified proportional hazards analysis. The sample is stratified by the variable that does not fit the proportionality assumption. Each stratum has its own baseline hazard. Therefore each stratum has a component that can vary over time differently from the other strata. The limitations of this strategy are the limitations of any stratified analysis. You can not assess the effect of the stratification variable on your outcome. Also, stratification is cumbersome if you have more than one or two variables that do not fit the proportionality assumption.

A third strategy is to switch your analysis to logistic regression. Because time is not taken into account in logistic regression models, the risks do not have to be proportional over time. The researchers assessing the factors associated with survival with AIDS in New York City (Section 8.5) switched their model from proportional hazards analysis to logistic analysis after they discovered the proportionality assumption "was seriously violated and could not be remedied through stratification." They created a dichotomous outcome variable: survival for fifteen months or longer (yes/no). They found several variables that were associated with survival at fifteen months. Although this solution avoided violating the proportionality assumption, one problem is that their results may be dependent on the cutoff they chose for their outcome. In other words, they may have found different factors associated with survival if they had chosen a cutoff of six or twenty-four months. This is especially problematic because the important research question is: What is associated with survival?, not: What is associated with survival at fifteen months? Also, any subjects who were lost to follow-up prior to fifteen months would have to be excluded from the analysis. Nevertheless, the researchers deserve credit for verifying the proportionality assumption and adapting their analysis; many authors do not report if and how they assessed the proportionality assumption.[80]

A fourth, and probably the best, strategy is to account for the lack of proportionality in the hazards. As explained in Section 10.11 this can be accomplished by setting up the model so that the relative hazard varies by period. You may also be able to transform the independent variable (e.g., polynomial transformation) so that it fits the proportionality assumption. Because these models are complex to set up, it would be best to consult with a biostatistician for help.

No matter what strategy you choose for your analysis, report to the reader how you assessed the assumption and whether it held. If it did not hold, don't feel discouraged. You have learned something, potentially important, about how the risk of your outcome changes over time under certain conditions.

✓ TIP

You can account for the lack of proportionality in a model by allowing the relative hazard to vary by period.

---

[80] Katz, M.H., Hauck, W.W. "Proportional hazards (Cox) regression." *J. Gen. Intern. Med.* 1993;8:702–11; Concato, J., Feinstein, A.R, Holford, T.R. "The risk of determining risk with multivariable models." *Ann. Intern. Med.* 1993;118:201–10.

11

Validation of Models

11.1 How can I validate my models?

Models rarely perform as well with new data as with the original data because the model maximizes the probability of obtaining the values of the original outcome data. Unless your new data are exactly the same as your original data, it would be surprising for a model based on maximizing the original data to perform as well on new data.

Although predictions based on the original cases will not be as accurate with new cases, the important question is how large is the decrement in performance. If the decrement is small, the model is said to be validated.

Rather than thinking of validation of models as a distinct activity, think of it as the extreme on a continuum of tests that you perform to evaluate the quality of your model. The continuum is shown in Figure 11.1.

The methods of validation are:

1. Collect new data.
2. Divide your existing data set:
   a. split-group,
   b. jackknife method,
   c. bootstrap.

Without question the best method of validating an empirical model is to collect more data and test the performance of the initial model with the new data. This was the case with the prognostic model for estimating survival for patients with primary melanoma (described in Section 2.1.C). The investigators found that four factors correctly classified the vital status (alive or dead) of 74% of the patients.

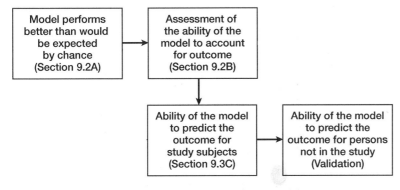

Figure 11.1. Continuum for assessing the quality of your model.

To validate their model, they studied the success of this four-variable model in predicting outcome among 142 patients who were diagnosed with primary melanoma in the same center in the two years following the enrollment of the initial sample. When applied to this new sample, the model correctly classified 69% of the patients, a relatively small decrement in performance from the original model.

Although testing the model with a second set of patients strengthens the validity of the model, it is not as strong a validation as testing the model on patients seen at a different center. The reason is that a model may not perform as well under a different set of circumstances (e.g., a different prevalence of disease, referral pattern, patient mix, clinician practice style or temporal changes). In the case of the melanoma prediction rule the only difference between the circumstances of the original and the second data set was the year of diagnosis, which makes it a somewhat less rigorous validation than if the investigators had enrolled subjects from a different institution.

With a split-group validation you randomly divide your data set into two parts – a derivation set (also called a training set) and a validation set (also called a confirmatory set). The parts can be equal halves or you can split the data set such that the derivation set is larger than the confirmatory set. You develop your model on the derivation set and then test it on the confirmatory set.

A split-group validation was used to test the validity of a model designed to predict recurrence of seizures.[81] The sample consisted of

> **▐▶ DEFINITION**
>
> With a *split-group* validation you randomly divide your data set into two parts – a derivation set and a validation set.

[81] Medical Research Council Antiepileptic Drug Withdrawal Study Group. "Prognostic index for recurrence of seizures after remission of epilepsy." *Br. Med. J.* 1993;306:1374–8.

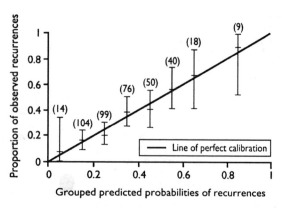

Figure 11.2. Comparison of the probability of predicted recurrences (probabilities are based on the model generated by the derivation set) to the observed probability of recurrences of seizures in the validation set. The bars show the confidence intervals for the predicted values and the dashes near the middle of the line show the mean predicted value. Reprinted with permission from Medical Research Council Antiepileptic Drug Withdrawal Study Group. "Prognostic index for recurrence of seizures after remission of epilepsy." *Br. Med. J.* 1993;306:1374–8. Copyright BMJ Publishing Group.

1,013 people who were free of seizures on medication for at least two years. The researchers were taking advantage of an existing data set to develop a prognostic model. Collection of additional data was not an option. Instead, the investigators randomly divided their existing sample into two parts, with 60% of their sample in the derivation set and 40% in the validation sample.

Using the derivation set they developed a proportional hazards model with eight prognostic factors. To validate the model they used it to estimate the probability of a recurrent seizure for each of the subjects in the validation data set. They grouped the estimated probabilities of seizure for the patients in the validation group into eight groups of increasing probability of recurrence. As shown in Figure 11.2, for each of the eight groups they compared the proportion of actual recurrences to that predicted by the model. The bars show the confidence intervals for the predicted values, and the dash near the middle of the line shows the mean predicted value. If the validation had been perfect, all dashes would fall exactly on the diagonal line. While the dashes are close to the diagonal line, the confidence intervals are broad, especially for those predicted values where the number of subjects (shown in parentheses) is small.

You will note that Figure 11.2 uses essentially the same technique as Figure 9.1. Figure 9.1 is also based on comparing predicted to observed probabilities. The difference is that in Figure 9.1 the predicted and observed probabilities are based on the same subjects. In Figure 11.2 the predicted probabilities are based on a model that was derived on a different group of subjects.

One final note about validating your model using a second sample or a split sample. Once a model has been validated, investigators will often combine the multiple samples or reunite the split sample for the final model. Investigators do this so that the larger sample size can give their final model tighter confidence intervals.

In cases where it is impractical to collect more data or split your sample, you may use a jackknife procedure (often called cross-validation). With a jackknife procedure you sequentially delete subjects from your data set, one at a time, and recompute your model with each subject missing once. This allows you to assess two things. First, you can assess the importance of any one subject to your results. A model that substantially changes with deletion of a single case is not valid because the results hinge on that one case. Second, once you drop a case, you can predict that subject's outcome from the remaining cases. This is done sequentially such that you are predicting the values of each subject using the rest of the subjects. In this sense, the jackknife is like a split-group validation: The split is the whole sample minus one case (the derivation set) versus the one case (the confirmatory set). When you have a relatively small sample, jackknife procedures are likely to be more sensible than splitting your sample. You should be aware that jackknife procedures are easy to do in multiple linear regression, but they are very computer time intensive in logistic and proportional hazards models.

> **▥➡ DEFINITION**
> ──────────
> With a *jackknife* procedure you sequentially delete subjects from your data set, one at a time, and recompute your model with each subject missing once.

The bootstrap procedure provides limited support of the validity of your model. With bootstrap procedures you take random samples of the subjects in your data set with replacement (meaning that after a case is chosen it becomes eligible to be chosen again). Thus, your random samples may include the same subject more than once whereas some subjects will not be included at all. Once the samples are drawn, you test the strength of the relationships found in your main model in the random samples. The results from these samples can be used to construct 95% confidence intervals by excluding the extreme 2.5% and 97.5% of values. If the confidence intervals are relatively narrow, you can feel more confident in your results.

For example, Hamberg and colleagues used logistic regression to create a model based on clinical and laboratory data that would

> **▥➡ DEFINITION**
> ──────────
> *Bootstrap* procedures take random samples of the subjects in your data set with replacement and average the results obtained from the multiple samples.

accurately predict cirrhosis among 303 alcohol-abusing men. Such a model would have clinical significance if it would decrease the need for liver biopsies. At a cutoff of 10% probability of having cirrhosis, the sensitivity and specificity of their model was 88%. They then tested their model using the same cutoff in a 1,000 samples drawn from their study population. The 95% confidence intervals for the sensitivity and specificity were 85%–91% and 85%–95% respectively.

Besides producing confidence intervals, bootstrap procedures produce mean coefficients and mean standard errors for your random samples. These confidence intervals and standard errors are likely to be more valid than those created from one simple model.[82]

The bootstrap procedure is a weaker test of the validity of a model than a split-group or a jackknife. This is because the 1,000 bootstrap samples of 303 subjects will have the majority of subjects in common. In contrast, a split sample and the jackknife procedures would have no subjects in common. Thus, in the strictest sense bootstrap does not fit the definition of validation.

The importance of validation varies with the goals of your study. Validation is rarely performed for studies identifying prognostic factors associated with a particular outcome while adjusting for confounders (Section 2.1.A). Your results will be judged primarily on the strength of your methods, the biologic plausibility of your results, and prior findings in this area. Other investigators may seek to replicate or refute your findings. In contrast, models predicting prognosis or diagnosis of disease (Sections 2.1.C and 2.1.D) are rarely published (at least not in the best journals) without validation.

The reason for the distinction is that models used to determine factors associated with a particular outcome do not need to be highly accurate. For example, while exercise is significantly associated with mortality, the decrease in mortality due to exercise is relatively small. You certainly would not try to predict a patient's life span based on knowing how much he or she exercises. But that's not the point. The point is that, in a population, exercising will result in increased longevity for the group as a whole. Improving risk factor profiles may have a substantial effect on the development of disease in a large population, even if the absolute effect for an individual is small. This is especially true if the disease and the risk factor are common.

---

[82] Readers interested in learning more about bootstrap techniques should see Efron, B., Tibshirania, R.J. *An Introduction to the Bootstrap.* New York: Chapman & Hall, 1993.

In contrast, with studies designed to predict diagnosis or prognosis, a high degree of certainty is required because you are using the model to predict for an individual patient. Clinicians are not likely to trust a model that has not been validated. (Even then, physicians are notorious for ignoring diagnostic algorithms, preferring instead their gut instinct; see Section 2.1.D.)

✓ **T I P**

Clinicians don't trust models that are not validated.

12

Special Topics

12.1 What if my data set has matched cases and controls?

Some research questions are more efficiently answered by matching cases to controls. In fact, much of traditional epidemiology is based on matched case–control studies where the investigators have assembled a group of people with the disease (the cases) and a group of people without the disease (the controls). Cases and controls are individually matched on a set of critical variables. (The key word here is individually matched. It is not a matched design if you choose a control group that as a whole is comparable to the group of cases).

What is the advantage of matching? By having controls that match your cases on potentially confounding variables you can answer the same question with a smaller sample than if you did not match. Why? Because you no longer have to adjust for the differences between the cases and the controls on the potentially confounding variables for which you matched (they are the same for each pair of cases and controls).

You may wonder why if matching allows you to eliminate confounding you would still need to do multivariable analysis. Indeed, if you were interested in assessing the impact of only one independent variable on the outcome, and had matched for all confounders of interest, you would not need to do multivariable analysis. Instead you would use a paired t test (for interval variables) or McNemar's test (for dichotomous variables). But, although matching eliminates confounding for the matched variables, there usually are other potential confounders for which the cases and controls are not matched. Also, remember that if you match on a particular variable, you can not assess the impact of that variable on the outcome.

✓ TIP

If you match on a particular variable, you can not assess the impact of that variable on the outcome.

The three models we have discussed in this book are not suitable for studies that individually match cases and controls because they do not link cases and controls to each other in the analysis. In other words, if you matched 100 cases with 100 controls, and analyzed them with the methods we have discussed thus far, the computer would not know which case went with which control. Therefore the analysis would not be individually matched.

To adapt the models to a matched sample, you could create a variable for each linked pair and adjust for these variables in your analysis. The problem is that this would result in your having many variables (the number of matched pairs in your study −1). Your analysis would have insufficient power to detect effects because no matter how large your sample size, you would have less than two subjects per variable. This is considerably less than the number of subjects needed per variable (Section 7.1).

Multivariable models are available that can incorporate individually matched data (Table 12.1). Repeated measures analysis of variance and conditional logistic regression are readily available and commonly used.[83] Although a modification of the proportional hazards model (i.e., marginal approach) is available, it is more complicated and requires the help of a biostatistician.[84]

A study of whether an appetite-suppressing drug causes primary pulmonary hypertension is a good example of the value of a matched multivariable model.[85] Primary pulmonary hypertension is a rare disease with a large number of suspected, but unproved, risk factors. Therefore the investigators matched 95 patients with primary pulmonary hypertension to 335 controls by age (within five years), gender, and the number of visits to the physician per year.

The authors found, using conditional logistic regression, that after adjustment for potential risk factors such as systemic hypertension, use of cocaine, and smoking status, use of appetite suppressants was

---

[83] For further information on repeated measures analysis of variance see Glantz, S.A., Slinker, B.K. *Primer of Applied Regression and Analysis of Variance*. New York: McGraw-Hill, 1990, pp. 391–452. For more on conditional logistic regression, see Hosmer, D.W., Lemeshow, S. *Applied Logistic Regression*. New York: Wiley, 1989, pp. 187–215.

[84] Lin, D.Y. "Cox regression analysis of multivariate failure time data: the marginal approach." *Stat. Med.* 1994;13:2233–47.

[85] Abenhaim, C., Moride, Y., Brenot, F., et al. "Appetite-suppressant drugs and the risk of primary pulmonary hypertension." *N. Engl. J. Med.* 1996; 335:609–16.

TABLE 12.1

Multivariable models for incorporating individually matched data

Interval outcome	Dichotomous outcome	Time to dichotomous outcome
Repeated measures analysis of variance	Conditional logistic regression	Marginal approach (for proportional hazards analysis)

significantly associated with an increased risk for primary pulmonary hypertension ($OR = 6.3$; 95% $CI = 3.0$–13.2). They also showed a dose–response relationship, with subjects who used appetite suppressants for more than three months having a risk of development of hypertension twenty-three times greater than that of persons who did not use appetite suppressants ($OR = 23.1$; 95% $CI = 6.9$–77.7).

12.2 What if my data set has repeated observations of outcome for the same individuals?

The multivariable methods that we have discussed thus far have assumed that you have observed the outcome of interest only once. However, multivariable models can incorporate repeated observations of outcome for the same individuals (Table 12.2).

With studies that have repeated observations for the same individuals, each case is its own control. Therefore, you need to individually link each case to itself, just as in matching designs. This is why the methods listed in Table 12.2 are similar to those listed in Table 12.1.

Repeated measures analysis of variance can analyze data with repeated observations and interval outcomes. Sometimes you may have a different number of repeated observations for different subjects (e.g., some subjects may have four examinations while other subjects have only three). Fortunately, unbalanced repeated measures models can incorporate different numbers of observations.[86]

[86] Jennrich, R.I., Schluchter, M.D. "Unbalanced repeated-measures models with structured covariance matrices." *Biometrics* 1986;42:805–20.

TABLE 12.2

Methods of analyzing data with repeated observations of outcome for the same individuals

Interval outcome	Dichotomous outcome	Time to dichotomous outcome
Repeated measures analysis of variance	Conditional logistic regression	Counting process Marginal approach
Change scores	Generalized estimation	
Slope	equations	

Another method for incorporating repeated observations of an interval outcome is to create a change score. A change score is the absolute or relative change of an outcome variable over the study period.

Consider the case of blood pressure, measured twice, six months apart. To determine the absolute change, you would simply subtract the baseline blood pressure measurement from the six-month blood pressure measurement. You would then use that new variable (change in blood pressure) as your outcome. In this way, you could observe how an independent variable, such as type of hypertension medication, affected the outcome without having to use a type of analysis that incorporates repeated observation of the same individuals.

Change scores can also be adapted to weigh relative changes more than absolute changes. This is done by dividing the change score by the baseline score. For example, with CD4 lymphocyte counts, a 100-cell change in six months would more likely be associated with progression of disease, if it reflected a drop from 200 cells to 100 cells than 1,200 cells to 1,100 cells. Both result in an absolute change of 100 cells but the relative change of the former is much larger ($100/200 = .5$) than the latter ($100/1,200 = .08$).

Change scores will not work when you have more than two observations. However, you can develop a measure of change over the course of the study period. This is usually done by plotting the observations for each case over time and determining the slope for each case.

> **⮞ DEFINITION**
>
> A *change score* is the absolute or relative change of your outcome variable over the study period.

> **✓ TIP**
>
> Slopes can be used to incorporate multiple measurements over time.

You can then use the slope as a dependent or independent variable. This works well for variables that increase (or decrease) in a linear fashion over time. Continuing with the example of serial CD4 lymphocyte counts, the slope of the CD4 count is often used by investigators as a measure of the rate of progression of disease over time because these counts decrease in a linear fashion (in the absence of therapy).[87]

Analogous to dividing a change score by the baseline value, you can divide the slope by its intercept. The result will be that changes that occur at high levels of your dependent variable will be weighted less than changes that occur at the lower values. This method was used by Riggs and colleagues to evaluate change in bone mineral density in their study of fluoride treatment of osteoporosis.[88]

An advantage of the use of slopes is that you don't lose a case if one measurement is missing or performed off schedule. To obtain a slope, you only need two points at any time. However, researchers usually will set a minimum of points needed to have a valid slope. (For example, Phillips and colleagues included only subjects who had at least five measurements of their CD4 count.) If the minimum number of measurements is not available, the case is considered missing.

For longitudinal designs that have repeated measures of a dichotomous outcome over time you can use an approach called generalized estimating equations. This method works particularly well when you have an outcome that is evaluated on multiple visits. For example, Hilton and colleagues studied the presence of oral candidiasis (yes/no) in HIV-infected transfusion recipients.[89] Transfusion recipients had oral examinations and CD4 counts performed every six months. CD4 counts were assessed at each visit. Using generalized estimation equations to model a logistic function, the authors demonstrated that having a low CD4 count at the current visit and oral candidiasis at a prior visit were associated with the presence of oral candidiasis.

Unlike the case with change scores, generalized estimation equations allow you to retain multiple outcomes for each participant. Repeated occurrences (or nonoccurrences) in the same individuals are

> ⏵ **DEFINITION**
>
> *Generalized estimation equations* allow you to account for the nonindependence of observations.

[87] Phillips, A.N., Lee, C.A., Elford, J., et al. "Serial CD4 lymphocyte counts and development of AIDS." *Lancet* 1991;337:389–92.

[88] Riggs, B.L., Hodgson, S.F., O'Fallon, W.M., et al. "Effect of fluoride treatment on the fracture rate in postmenopausal women with osteoporosis." *N. Engl. J. Med.* 1990;322:802–9.

[89] Hilton, J.F., Donegan, E., Katz, M.H., et al. "Development of oral lesions in human immunodeficiency virus-infected transfusion recipients and hemophiliacs." *Am. J. Epidemiol.* 1997;14:44–55.

168   SPECIAL TOPICS

not independent. In general, subjects who have an outcome once are more likely to have that same outcome again; conversely, subjects who have not had an outcome for a period of time are less likely to have that outcome in the future. The three methods we have discussed in this book – multiple linear regression, logistic regression, and proportional hazards – assume independent observations. One of the strengths of generalized estimation equations is that they allow you to account for the nonindependence of observations (multiple examinations of the same people) by adjusting the significance levels to account for the lack of independence of the observations.

This technique has tremendous flexibility. All subjects do not need to have the same number of visits. Also, your analysis can include independent variables measured only once (such as gender) as well as variables measured on multiple occasions (CD4 count). It gives you much greater power to find an effect in studies that have a small number of subjects but a large number of observations. In the study of HIV-infected transfusion recipients there were only 154 subjects but there were over a 1,000 oral examinations. Setting up generalized estimation equations correctly is challenging, and, if your data require this approach, I recommend that you consult a biostatistician, as well as the references listed.[90]

For studies of time to a dichotomous outcome, where you have repeated outcomes, it is possible to generalize the proportional hazards model. Two generalizations that are used are the counting process formulation and modeling marginal distributions. These generalizations are used in situations when the repeated outcome is clearly a new episode and not a recurrence of the first episode. The reason I emphasize not a recurrence is that the factors associated with recurrence of a disease are usually different from the factors associated with that disease. For example, in a model of development of breast cancer, you wouldn't include women who already had breast cancer. Whereas family history and late childbearing have the strongest association with development of breast cancer, stage of disease, hormone receptors, and histologic grade are the strongest risk factors for recurrence of breast cancer. Of course, it is perfectly sensible to model time to recurrence; but this does not involve repeated outcomes; there is only one outcome (first recurrence).

---

[90] Zeger, S.L., Liang, K.Y. "Longitudinal data analysis using generalized linear models." *Biometrika* 1986;73:13–22; Zegler, S.L., Liang, K.Y. "Longitudinal data analysis for discrete and continuous outcomes." *Biometrics* 1986;42:121–30.

For those diseases for which it is sensible to speak of a second distinct episode, where the risk factors for a second episode may be similar to the risk factors for a first episode, the counting process adaptation of proportional hazards analysis may work well. For example, Hooton and colleagues were interested in studying urinary tract infections in young women.[91] With urinary tract infections, patients can have a second (or third, etc.) episode after a "cured" first episode. Therefore, Hooton and colleagues included repeat episodes in their analysis, which increased the power of their study.

While a second episode of a urinary infection can occur after a cured episode, repeated episodes in the same person are not independent observations. Why? Because the causes of urinary track infections are likely to be more similar in repeated episodes in the same person than in separate episodes in different people. So, to include repeated episodes, your model must account for the partial dependence of repeated episodes in the same person.

For example, to include women with multiple urinary tract infections Hooton and colleagues used the counting process formulation of proportional hazards analysis to adjust for the correlations within subjects. The mechanics of this method, as well as the mechanics of modeling marginal distributions – the other method for handling multiple outcomes in the same individuals – are beyond the scope of this book. For guidance, see the references[92] and your biostatistician. If you do not wish to tackle this methodically challenging task and the number of people with multiple episodes is small, consider counting only the first episode in your analysis.

✓ **T I P**

You must use special methods to deal with outcomes that can occur in more than one body part in the same person because the observations are not independent.

12.3 What if my outcome can occur in more than one body part in the same person?

Clinical researchers in the fields of ophthalmology, orthopedics, and dentistry have a distinct advantage over cardiologists, neurologists, and hepatologists. What is it? While humans have only one heart, one

[91] Hooton, T.M., Scholes, D., Hughes, J.P., et al. "A prospective study of risk factors for symptomatic urinary tract infection in young women." *N. Engl. J. Med.* 1996; 335:468–74.

[92] Anderson, P.K., Gill, R.D. "Cox's regression model for counting processes: a large sample study." *Ann. Stat.* 1982;10:1100–20; Wei, L.J., Lin, D.Y., Weissfeld, L. "Regression analysis of multivariate incomplete failure time data by modeling marginal distributions." *J. Am. Stat. Assoc.* 1989;84:1065–73; Lin, D.Y., Wei, L.J. "The robust inference for the Cox proportional hazards model." *J. Am. Stat. Assoc.* 1989;84:1074–78.

SPECIAL TOPICS

TABLE 12.3

Methods of analyzing data for outcomes that can occur in more than one body part in the same person.

Interval outcome	Dichotomous outcome	Time to dichotomous outcome
Repeated measures analysis of variance	Generalized estimating equations	Marginal approach

brain, and one liver, we have two eyes, most of our joints in duplicate, and thirty-two or so teeth. In those fields with duplicate organs, it is possible to follow (or assess) a single subject and have multiple observations. However, as is the case with outcomes that are observed more than once in a single subject (Section 12.2), you must use special methods to deal with outcomes that can occur in more than one body part in the same person. The reason is the same: The observations are not independent. Two knees in the same person are more likely to have the same outcome than two knees in different people. Multivariable methods of analyzing data for outcomes that can occur in more than one body part are shown in Table 12.3.

In a study of the relationship of vitamin D to development of osteoarthritis of the knee, the investigators used the fact that their participants had two knees to their advantage.[93] Although the Framingham study consists of over 5,000 subjects, only 556 participants had x-rays of their knees and assessments of their vitamin D intake and serum levels. Therefore, the investigators needed to maximize their statistical power. They did this by looking at both knees. They used generalized estimation equations to adjust for the correlation between knees in the same person.

The investigators found that vitamin D was associated with progression of osteoarthritis. Question: Does adjustment for the dependence between the two knees eliminate the bias that osteoarthritis in one knee may cause osteoarthritis in the other knee due to changes in

---

[93] McAlindon, T.E., Felson, D.T., Zhang, Y., et al. "Relation of dietary intake and serum levels of vitamin D to progression of osteoarthritis of the knee among participants in the Framingham study." *Ann. Intern. Med.* 1996;125:353–9.

the person's gait? No. The adjustment only deals with the likelihood that vitamin D will affect two knees of the same person more similarly than two knees belonging to different persons. What should the investigators do to eliminate the bias due to changes in gait caused by a bad knee? Censor the good knee at the time that the other knee develops arthritis. This is what the investigators did.

The marginal approach for the proportional hazards model can also be used when the outcome can occur to more than one body part in the same person. For example, in a study of complications after breast implantation most women had bilateral implants.[94] Some had multiple implants in the same breast. The investigators therefore performed follow-up of each breast implant until a complication occurred, the implant was removed, or the end of follow-up occurred. However, they used a marginal approach because the time until complication was correlated for implants from the same women. Notice the differences and similarities between this example and that of the repeated urinary tract infections (Section 12.2). In this study the women had multiple implants, whereas in the urinary tract infection study, subjects only have one urinary track. But, in both cases, it is possible to speak of repeated outcomes in the same person. To analyze repeated outcomes in the same person, we must use methods that take into account the correlations between these repeated outcomes.

I hope you take away from this section and Section 12.2 that:

- It is possible to incorporate multiple outcomes for the same individuals.
- When you have multiple outcomes for the same individuals you must use methods that adjust for the lack of independence of the outcomes.
- The methods for adjusting for the lack of independence are complicated, and you should consult a biostatistician to help you carry them out.

12.4 What if the independent variable changes value during the course of the study?

Let's say that over the course of a longitudinal study a subject's value changes on an independent variable. This may happen because the patient quits (or starts) a habit such as smoking, begins a new medicine,

---

[94] Gabriel, S.E., Woods, J.E., O'Fallon, W.M., et al. "Complications leading to surgery after breast implantation." *N. Engl. J. Med.* 1997;336:677–82.

or develops a new symptom or illness. How can you deal with this in your analysis? The answer is that within proportional hazards analysis you can create time-dependent variables. These variables change value at a particular point in time. So, instead of having a variable such as smoking at baseline (yes/no), you create a time-dependent variable, where each subject is 0 (nonsmoker) or 1 (smoker) at a particular point of survival time.

In the simplest case, time-dependent variables change their value only once (e.g., a nonsmoker starts to smoke – the variable is 0, 0, 0, at several points in time before the subject begins smoking and then the variable changes value to 1 at the time the subject begins smoking and remains 1 for the remainder of the observational time). It is also possible to construct time-dependent variables that change their value back and forth multiple times (reflecting what sometimes happens when smokers try to quit). Time-dependent variables need not be dichotomous; that is, the variable may take the value of an interval measure, such as blood pressure, at each point that it is measured.

While the interpretation of time-dependent variables can be complicated, their construction is easy. You need to look up the exact formatting in your statistical package, but in general, the package will have a special designation for time-dependent variables. You tell the computer when (in study time) each subject changes value on the variable.

12.5 What are the advantages and disadvantages of time-dependent covariates?

The advantage of time-dependent covariates is that you can incorporate important events that occur during the course of the study. For example, Mayne and colleagues wanted to determine if depression shortened survival of HIV-infected men.[95] Their subjects were part of a longitudinal study that began in 1984 with more than seven years of follow-up. The simplest design for answering this question would be to measure depression in 1984 and then follow subjects longitudinally for mortality. The problem with this design is that depression may not be present initially (in 1984) but may develop subsequently. Using depression at baseline only will weaken your study (because people who

---

[95] Mayne, T.J., Vittinghoff, E., Chesney, M.A., Barrett, D.C., Coates, T.J. "Depressive effect and survival among gay and bisexual men infected with HIV." *Arch. Intern. Med.* 1996;156:2233–8.

become depressed six months after baseline will not be considered depressed in the analysis, even though this may affect their mortality). Second, using depression only at baseline decreases your power because relatively few persons will be classified as depressed at one time. Third, a single instance of a participant being rated as depressed might not affect mortality, since it might reflect only a short episode of depression, rather than a more chronic condition.

To overcome these issues, the researchers created a time-dependent variable that took the value of the proportion of visits at which the person was depressed. So for each visit (subjects were interviewed every six months) the variable had a value between 0% and 100% (of visits to date) at which the person was depressed. They found that depression was associated with a higher rate of mortality. They also created time-dependent variables that represented each subject's actual score on the depression index at each visit. The results were similar.

The depression measure was not the only variable that changed value over the course of this study. The subjects' immune function also changed value as patients progressed. The investigators therefore created time-dependent covariates that represented the subjects' CD4 counts, as well as other measures of immune function. They found that depression increased the risk of death, even with adjustment for changes in immune function. This would suggest that the mechanism of depression on mortality is not mediated by more rapid immune function decline (within the limits of the investigators' ability to measure it). This analysis also weakens an "effect–cause" hypothesis (that participants became depressed because they learned of their CD4 count results), since the analysis adjusts for recent CD4 counts.

Another advantage of time-dependent covariates is that they do not have to fit the proportionality assumption (Section 10.10). The reason is that they incorporate time and therefore do not have to be independent of time.

The disadvantages of time-dependent covariates are less obvious than the advantages. The two major ones are: overadjustment and decreased usefulness of the model for clinicians.

Adjusting for prognostic markers that are on the pathway to your outcome may prevent you from identifying the effect you are investigating (overadjustment). Let's go back to the example of depression and mortality in HIV-infected persons. Assume that the overall finding is accurate, that is, that depression increases mortality. But, let's assume that the mechanism by which this happens is that depression leads to worsening immune function, which, in turn, leads to more opportunistic infections and death. If this is the case, then including time-dependent variables measuring immune function will eliminate the effect you are trying to substantiate. Depression will not be associated with mortality because adjusting for changes in immune function will eliminate the effect. In comparison, if you adjust only for immune function at baseline you would not eliminate the effect.

The use of time-dependent covariates may also decrease the value of your models for clinicians. The reason is that clinicians must advise their patients based on information they have at the time they are counseling the patient. A clinician can't know how a risk factor will change in the future. It would be confusing to a patient to counsel them on their risk of heart attack in case they *were* to develop hypertension at a particular time in the future.

With time-dependent models it is important to include only events that have occurred before the outcome. Remember that an advantage of a longitudinal design compared to a cross-sectional one is that a longitudinal study is more likely to support causality. That's because if the outcome is not yet present (at least, as best as can be measured), the chance that the "outcome" causes the "risk factor" (i.e., effect–cause) is much less likely. (Remember, in a cross-sectional study you are measuring risk factors and outcomes at the same time.) With time-dependent variables, you are including factors that are more proximal to outcome than baseline measurements. Thus, effect–cause becomes a greater danger. One way to deal with this issue is to "lag" the time-dependent measure substantially before the outcome (but still after the baseline).

> ✓ **TIP**
>
> With time-dependent covariates include only events that have occurred before the outcome.

A lag for time-dependent variables was used by the investigators to see if depression would still be associated with mortality if the depression measure was lagged by periods of one, two, and three years from the outcome. With these time lags, depression was still associated with mortality, supporting the hypothesis that depression increases mortality, and weakening the case for the alternative hypothesis that depression reflects worsening health status.

12.6 What if the frequency of my outcome is really low over time (rare disease)?

For outcomes that occur rarely over time ($<5\%$), proportional hazards analysis is not valid. Instead, use Poisson regression. Although the mechanics of Poisson regression are beyond the scope of this book,

> ✓ **TIP**
>
> Use Poisson regression for rare outcomes.

the output and interpretation is quite similar. Poisson regression will provide you with coefficients, relative risks (based on comparing the incidence rates), and 95% confidence intervals.

Poisson regression was used to examine the risk of stroke due to pregnancy.[96] In the study catchment area there were 1,051,113 women of reproductive age. The investigators found 31 strokes during 8,011,852 weeks of exposure time (exposure time was the pregnancy and the six-week post-partum period) and 223 strokes during 101,303,016 weeks of nonexposure time (not pregnant). Thus in the study there was a total of 254 strokes in 109,314,868 weeks (incidence of .01 strokes per hundred women-years). Despite this rare outcome, Poisson regression showed a significantly elevated risk of stroke associated with pregnancy (relative risk for pregnancy was 2.4; 95% CI = 1.6–3.6), after adjustment for age and race.

To learn more about how to perform Poisson regression see listed references[97] or consult a biostatistician.

12.7 What are classification and regression trees (CART) and should I use them?

Classification and regression trees (CART), also known as recursive partitioning, are techniques for separating (partitioning) your subjects into distinct subgroups based on the outcome.

The technique is easiest to follow visually. In Figure 12.1, you see an algorithm for assessing the risk of heart attack that was developed using CART.[98] The algorithm is based on 1,379 patients, of whom 259 (19%) had a heart attack. The investigators assessed the diagnostic ability of fifty variables, including patients' history, physical examination, and electrocardiogram results.

CART attempts to divide the sample into subgroups that have as many patients with the outcome (e.g., heart attack) in one group (high

---

[96] Kittner, S.J., Stern, B.J., Feeser, B.R., et al. "Pregnancy and the risk of stroke." *N. Engl. J. Med.* 1996;335:768–74.

[97] Kleinbaum, D.G., Kupper, L.L., Muller, K.E. *Applied Regression Analysis and Other Multivariable Methods* (2nd ed.). Boston: PWS-Kent, 1988, pp. 497–512; Gardner, W., Mulvey, E.P., Shaw, E. "Regression analyses of counts and rates: Poisson, overdispersed Poisson, and negative binomial models." *Psych. Bull.* 1995;118:392–404.

[98] Goldman, L., Cook, E.F., Brand, D.A., et al. "A computer protocol to predict myocardial infarction in emergency department patients with chest pain." *N. Engl. J. Med.* 1988;318:797–803.

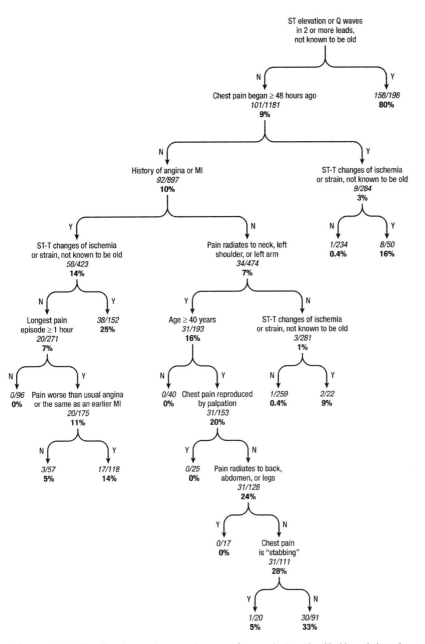

Figure 12.1. Classification and regression tree for predicting the likelihood that the patient has a myocardial infarction. The data are from Goldman, L., et al. "A computer protocol to predict myocardial infarction in emergency department patients with chest pain." *N. Engl. J. Med.* 1988;318:797–803. The figure is adapted from Lee, T.H., et al. "Ruling out acute myocardial infarction." *N. Engl. J. Med.* 1991;324:1239–46. Copyright ©1991 Massachusetts Medical Society. All rights reserved.

risk) and as few patients with the outcome in the other group (low risk). You can see that at the first branch point of Figure 12.1 (ST elevation or Q waves in two or more leads, not known to be old), CART separates the sample into two groups with very different probabilities of heart attack: 80% and 9%. At the next branch point (chest pain began ≥48 hours ago), the sample is also separated into two groups with different probabilities of outcome (10% vs. 3%), although this difference is not as large as the difference in the first branch point. CART will continue partitioning, selecting from the fifty candidate variables, until it reaches a point where it is no longer possible to partition the sample into subgroups with distinctly different risks of outcome. If your CART model partitions your sample into subgroups where the risks are not sufficiently distinct, you can prune your tree back.

What advantage does CART have over other multivariable techniques? It is similar to forward stepwise logistic regression in that you are estimating a dichotomous outcome by sequentially choosing the strongest risk factors for your outcome. In fact, forward stepwise logistic regression produces a similar answer as CART when applied to these heart attack prediction data.[99]

> The major difference between CART and forward logistic regression is that with CART one branch can have different risk factors for outcome than a different branch.

The major difference between CART and forward multiple logistic regression is that with CART one branch can have different risk factors for outcome than a different branch. With multiple logistic regression your risk factors are for your entire sample, not one branch of it. For this reason, CART is better suited to data where there are interactions (because with interactions a variable may be important for only a portion of the sample) (see Sections 1.4, 8.3, 9.9, and 10.8).

An advantage of diagnostic trees is that compared with multiple logistic regression they more closely reflect how physicians make decisions. Certain pieces of information take you down a particular diagnostic path; you seek more information to prove or disprove that you are on the right path. Most clinicians do not, in their mind, total up all the information, positive and negative, and make a decision.

Having said that, clinicians have shown no greater willingness to adopt this decision rule than that of Pozen and colleagues. When the authors attached their prediction tree to the back of the patient data forms in their own hospital, physicians looked at it in only 46% of the

---

[99] See the bible of CART: Breiman, L., Friedman, J.H., Olshen, R.A., Stone, C.J. *Classification and Regression Trees.* Pacific Grove, CA: Wadsworth & Brooks, 1984, p. 189.

cases; in the 115 cases in which the prediction rule was used, it changed the triage decision only once. Moreover, the likelihood of using the rule decreased with increased level of physician training (i.e., interns used it more than residents who used it more than attendings). This is despite the fact that the decision model shown in Figure 12.1 was shown to perform better than physicians at university and community hospitals when tested prospectively.

One disadvantage of the chest pain model is the large number of variables it includes. One widely used algorithm that was developed using CART predicts whether or not a patient has an ankle fracture based on only three variables.[100] The model, referred to as the Ottawa ankle rules, has a sensitivity of 100% for predicting fracture. Therefore, patients who are negative on the decision rule do not need to be sent for an x-ray film. This saves a great deal of money and time for the patient. The lower specificity of the model (50%) is not a major problem because at one time practically all patients with an ankle injury would have received an x-ray.

Because of their convenience and high sensitivity, the Ottawa ankle rules have received much wider acceptance than the heart attack prediction models. This should not, however, be taken as a negative reflection on heart attack prediction models. It is not surprising that it takes more variables to accurately predict a heart attack than a broken ankle, and that even with a large number of variables, there is greater uncertainty in the prediction of a heart attack than a broken ankle. It does highlight, however, that clinicians are more likely to adapt diagnostic rules that are simple and have high sensitivity.

12.8 How can I get best use of my biostatistician?

All biostatisticians are not alike. Some are primarily interested in developing new methods of analyzing data (data at the service of methods). Others are interested in using methods for improving the analysis of the data (methods at the service of data). In general, you will do better if you have the latter type of biostatistician, although we wouldn't have so many useful statistical techniques if it were not for the former type.

[100] Stiell, I.G., Greenberg, G.H., McKnight, D., et al. "Decision rules for the use of radiography in acute ankle injuries: Refinement and prospective validation." *JAMA* 1993;269:1127–32; Stiell, I.G., McKnight, R.D., Greenberg, G.H., et al. "Implementation of the Ottawa ankle rules." *JAMA* 1994;271:827–32.

Just as it helps to know more about your car in dealing with car mechanics, the more you know about your research project, and the statistical issues surrounding it, the more helpful your biostatistician will be to you. It is unlikely that most biostatisticians will get to know your data as well as you do. Use them as consultants.

At the design phase of your project, review with them the possible design options for your study. For complicated designs, ask their help on the power calculations. Once you have assembled your data set review it thoroughly before you seek consultation. (It will be more efficient and save you money!) All analyses begin with univariate and bivariate analyses. Follow the steps outlined in Chapter 14. In the process of analyzing your data, you may encounter problems: skewed distributions, nonlinear relationships, multicollinearity, and missing data. Review the parts of this book dealing with these issues. Think about their clinical implications and the possible solutions. Ask yourself what are the possible options for the situation and what the pros and cons are for each option. Then review this with your biostatistician.

12.9 How do I choose which software package to use?

Almost all of the popular statistical packages (SAS, SPSS, BMDP, STATA, S-PLUS) perform the same types of analyses. The best one to choose will likely depend on what others in your research group use. Programming questions invariably arise and it is always helpful to have other users nearby.

As with foreign languages, some statistical packages are harder to learn than others, but once you know one it is easier to learn others. While I have not performed any formal polling, most medical researchers uses SAS. On the one hand, SAS is somewhat more difficult to learn than the others, in part, because the manuals are poorly organized and confusing. On the other hand, SAS is more flexible and powerful than most of the others. The flexibility is particularly important for longitudinal studies, where you have multiple observations of the same person. SAS also allows you to write your own statistical programs but it also costs more than some of the others.

Some packages are particularly good at certain functions. S-PLUS is dramatically increasing in popularity because it has fantastic graphing capabilities. SUDAAN is often chosen for data sets that require adjustment for cluster effects or standardization to a broader population.

13

Publishing Your Study

13.1 How much information about how I constructed my multivariable models should I put in the Methods section?

The editors of the major biomedical journals have developed guidelines on how much detail of the statistical analysis to include in manuscripts. While the guidelines are general, the editors articulate an important rule of thumb: "Describe statistical methods with enough detail to enable a knowledgeable reader with access to the original data to verify the reported results."[101]

Although that goal is important, anyone who has performed statistical analysis knows that it would be impossible to include every detail of the analysis in a manuscript. Imagine writing: "for each independent variable we assessed whether there was any difference in outcome between the don't know category and the missing category" or "for one variable, we found that there was a somewhat increased frequency of outcome in the don't know versus the missing category, so we ..." I think you get the idea. Research requires thousands of decisions. The readers rely on you to make the right ones. It is your responsibility, however, to report on the important choices you made, especially those that influence the results.

Published articles and journals differ in how they organize the information in the Methods section. I prefer dividing the Methods section into review of how subjects were enrolled (Subjects), what

---

[101] International Committee of Medical Journal Editors. "Uniform requirements for manuscripts submitted to biomedical journals." *Ann. Intern. Med.* 1997; 126:36–47; Begg, C., Cho, M., Eastwood, S., et al. "Improving the quality of reporting of randomized controlled trials: the CONSORT statement." *JAMA* 1996; 276:637–9.

interventions were used or how data were acquired (Procedures), how the variables were coded (Measures), and how the data were analyzed (Statistical analysis). But some published articles group all of the information under a general heading of Methods. Before writing this section for your manuscript, consult a recent issue of the journal to which you plan to submit your paper; you will get a sense of the journal's preferences. At a minimum, include a description of the following in your methods section:

1. The population from which your subjects was chosen and your method of choosing them (e.g., probability sample of households in low income census tracts, consecutive sample of patients presenting to a specialty clinic with sinusitis).
2. If any sampled subjects were excluded and if so why (e.g., insufficient blood sample).
3. Response rate, including differences between persons who participated in your study and those who did not. (Some journals prefer that this information be reported in the Results section.)
4. Nature of intervention (e.g., patients were randomized to one of three arms of drug therapy) if applicable.
5. How data were acquired (e.g., interviews, matches with registries).
6. How your independent and dependent variables were chosen and measured.
7. How your independent and dependent variables are categorized in the analysis (e.g., nominal, multiple dichotomous variables).
8. What bivariate statistics you used (e.g., chi-square statistics for categorical variables, t tests for interval variables).
9. What type of multivariable model you used (e.g., multiple linear regression, conditional logistic regression).
10. How you dealt with missing data.
11. What independent variables were eligible for inclusion in the model (e.g., all variables in your Table 1, those independent variables associated with the outcome at $P < .15$).
12. If you used a variable selection procedure, state type (e.g., forward, backward) and what the inclusion/exclusion criteria were (e.g., $P < .10$).
13. If you had censored observations, when you censored them (e.g., alternative outcomes, date of the end of the observation period).
14. How you tested the linearity assumption.
15. How you tested the proportionality assumption (for proportional hazards model).

16. Whether you tested for interactions and, if so, how.
17. What statistical software you used. (The reason for this is that some packages differ in their computational methods for certain statistics.)
18. Whether *P* values were one- or two-tailed.

Within the Methods section, my preference is to report 1–3 in the Subjects subsection, 4 and 5 in the Procedures subsection, 6 and 7 in the Measures section, and 8–18 in the Statistical analysis subsection, but, journals and reviewers vary in their preferences.

13.2 Do I need to cite a statistical reference for my choice of multivariable models?

If you are doing a standard linear or logistic regression analysis it is unnecessary to provide a citation. Some researchers provide a citation for proportional hazards regression. It is always the same citation:

> Cox, D.R. "Regression models and life tables." *J. R. Stat. Soc.* 1972; 34:187–220.

I would predict in five years we will no longer cite Cox's paper (despite the great contribution he made), because the field will be sufficiently comfortable with the model. Some of the techniques I discussed in the Special Topics chapter, such as methods for adjusting for multiple outcomes in the same individual, should also be cited.

13.3 Which parts of my multivariable analysis should I report in the Results section?

As with the question of what to include in the Methods section, there are no absolute rules on what results to report in your published paper.

Unless there are no missing data, you should report the N for each analysis. For multiple linear regression models, most investigators report the regression coefficients (standardized or unstandardized, but not both), the standard errors of the coefficients, and the statistical significance levels of the coefficients. As a test of how well the model accounts for the outcome, most researchers report the adjusted R^2.

For logistic regression and proportional hazards analysis, even though the coefficients are similar to those from linear regression, they are not generally reported. Instead, report the odds ratio or relative hazard and the 95% confidence interval. The latter incorporates

TABLE 13.1

Relative risk of cardiovascular disease among current users of conjugated estrogen alone or with progestin as compared with nonusers, 1978 to 1992.*

HORMONE USE	PERSON-YEARS	MAJOR CORONARY DISEASE			STROKE (ALL TYPES)		
		NO. OF CASES	RELATIVE RISK (95% CI)		NO. OF CASES	RELATIVE RISK (95% CI)	
			Age Adjusted	Multivariate Adjusted[†]		Age Adjusted	Multivariate Adjusted[†]
Never used	304,744	431	1.0		270	1.0	
Currently used							
Estrogen alone	82,626	47	0.45 (0.34–0.60)	0.60 (0.43–0.83)	74	1.13 (0.88–1.46)	1.27 (0.95–1.69)
Estrogen with progestin	27,161	8	0.22 (0.12–0.41)	0.39 (0.19–0.78)	17	0.74 (0.45–1.20)	1.09 (0.66–1.80)

* CI denotes confidence interval.

† The analysis was adjusted for age (in five-year categories), time (in two-year categories), age at menopause (in two-year categories), body-mass index (in quintiles), diabetes (yes or no), high blood pressure (yes or no), high cholesterol level (yes or no), cigarette smoking (never, formerly, or currently [1 to 14, 15 to 24, or 25 or more cigarettes per day]), past oral-contraceptive use (yes or no), parental history of myocardial infarction before the age of 60 years (yes or no), and type of menopause (natural or surgical).

Reprinted with permission from Grodstein, F., et al. "Postmenopausal estrogen and progestin use and the risk of cardiovascular disease." *N. Engl. J. Med.* 1996;335:453–61. Copyright © 1996 Massachusetts Medical Society. All rights reserved.

be less helpful to future researchers. For example, if someone was doing a meta-analysis on the effect of past oral-contraceptive use (a variable that has been inconsistently related to outcomes such as coronary disease and stroke) they wouldn't learn anything from the table. You don't know whether oral contraceptives are or are not related to the outcomes in this study.

Finally, when evaluating a published report, one feels greater confidence if the independent variables operate in ways you would expect them to based on prior research. For example, if the investigators reported that cigarette smoking was related to coronary artery disease and stroke it would give you confidence that their model was sound. Conversely, if smoking was not related to these outcomes you would worry about the validity of their model.

All this being said, demands and cost of journal space are likely to dictate more presentations of data like Table 13.1. With large models, and multiple independent variables, it is hard to show all the results. One solution to this dilemma is gaining in popularity: Investigators inform readers where they can obtain the full analysis (usually by writing to the authors or through a national repository). This seems a good balance between publishing extensive tables and having results available to the public.

> ✓ **T I P**
>
> If you are unable to publish your full analysis, send your detailed results to a national repository.

14

Summary: Steps for Constructing a Multivariable Model

Step 1. Based on the type of outcome variable you have use Table 3.1 to determine the type of multivariable model to perform.

Step 2. Perform univariate statistics to understand the distribution of your independent and outcome variables. Assess for implausible values, significant departures from normal distribution of interval variables, gaps in values, and outliers (Section 5.7).

Step 3. Perform bivariate analysis of your independent variables against your outcome variable.

Step 4. If you have any nominal independent variables transform them into multiple dichotomous ("dummied") variables (Section 4.2).

Step 5. Assess whether your data fit the assumptions of your multi-variable model (linearity, normal distribution, equal variance) on a bivariate basis (Chapter 5). Transform or group any variables that show significant bivariate departures from the assumptions of your model (Sections 5.4, 5.5, 5.7, and 5.8).

Step 6. Run a correlation matrix. If any pair of independent variables are correlated at >.90 (multicollinearity) decide which one to keep and which one to exclude. If any pair of variables are correlated at .80 to .90 consider dropping one (Chapter 6).

Step 7. Assess how much missing data you will have in your multi-variable analysis. Choose a strategy for dealing with missing cases from Table 8.6.

Step 8. Perform the analysis. Choose a variable selection technique most suited to your study (Sections 8.9 and 8.11).

Step 9. Review the multivariable correlation matrix to assess for multi-collinearity. If you have evidence of serious multicollinearity, delete a variable (Chapter 6).

Step 10. Assess whether your model accounts for outcome better than would be expected by chance (e.g., F test, likelihood ratio test) (Section 9.2.A).

Step 11. Perform an assessment of the fit of your model (e.g., adjusted R^2, Hosmer–Lemeshow test) (Section 9.2.B) or its ability to predict the outcome for study subjects (e.g., sensitivity, c index) (Section 9.2.C).

Step 12. Assess the strength of your individual covariates in estimating outcome (Section 9.3).

Step 13. Evaluate whether your data fit the multivariable assumptions of your model (Chapter 10). Use regression diagnostics to test how well your model fits your data on a multivariable level (Sections 10.1–10.6). For proportional hazards models, be sure that the proportionality assumption is met (Sections 10.10–10.12).

Step 14. Decide whether to include interaction terms in your model (Sections 1.4, 8.3, 9.9, and 10.8).

Step 15. Consider whether it would be possible to validate your model (Chapter 11).

Step 16. Publish your results in the *New England Journal of Medicine* and be the envy of your friends and colleagues.

Step 17. Send me a reprint so I'll know that the above worked. (Also send questions or suggestions for future editions.)

Mitchell Katz, MD
Director of Health
101 Grove Street, Room 308
San Francisco, CA 94102-4593

SUMMARY: STEPS FOR CONSTRUCTING A MULTIVARIABLE MODEL

Index